Your Ideal Hawaii Health

Why people in Hawaii are so Healthy and Happy

Tyler Mercier
Chris Mercier

ISBN: **1505390214**
ISBN-13: **978-1505390216**

PO Box 1029
Kailua-Kona, Hawaii 96745

Library of Congress Control Number: **2014-922949**

Photos, art, layout, and design by authors.

<u>Limits of Liability and Disclaimer</u>
This book is based on the experiences of the authors in Hawaii. It is not intended to replace the advice from medical and health professionals. The authors shall not be held liable for any incidental or consequential damages in connection with or arising out of the use of information contained in this book.

CONTENTS

INTRODUCTION

Since moving to Hawaii, we have had fantastic improvement in our health and fitness. Yet it was a mystery to us why so many people living in Hawaii are healthier, happier, and live longer. We wanted to know the secret of health and fitness in Hawaii so we would not change something in our life that would reverse our progress.

Hawaii was ranked the most "healthy" in the nation by the United Health Foundation based on the state's low cancer deaths, low cardiovascular deaths, low rate of diabetes, low rate of obesity, high levels of physical activity, low rate of preventable hospitalizations, and low numbers of smokers.[1] Hawaii has the lowest mortality rate in the nation. Hawaii also has the lowest rate of depression among seniors in the nation and the lowest rate of obesity among seniors.[1] Best of all, according to the Gallup Healthways Well Being Index, Hawaii is ranked as one of the "happiest" states in the US.[2]

Why are people who live in Hawaii thinner, healthier, and happier than people who live elsewhere in the US? What is it about Hawaii that makes people live so long? We wanted to know the answer to these questions and so did our friends.

Our research uncovered numerous reasons why people improve their health and lose weight in Hawaii. Many of the things we learned that make the Hawaiian Islands a healthy place to live can be copied anywhere. We wish we had known these things when were younger and lived on the mainland. It would have saved us from years of being obese and stressed out.

This book describes what we learned from our extensive research about how the ocean, sunshine, food, activities, and slow pace of life in Hawaii improve health. We cite the latest research and tell about our experiences while making dramatic changes in our diet and lifestyle to achieve our health goals.

INTRODUCTION

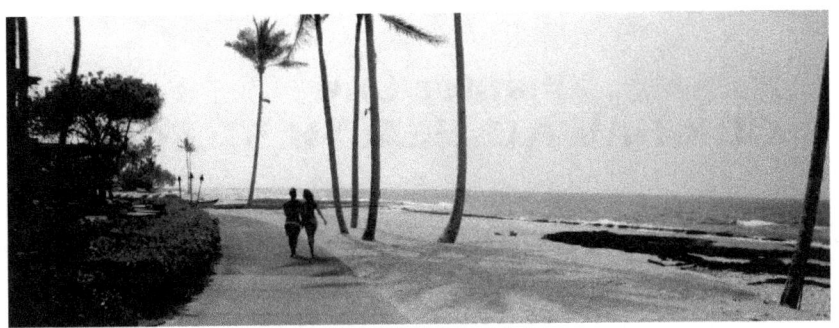

References

1. United Health Foundation, website:
http://www.americashealthrankings.org
last accessed 12/1/14.
2. Gallup Healthways, State of Hawaii Well-Being:
2013 State, Community, and Congressional
District Analysis, online report available on
http://www.healthways.com.

Chapter One
OUR HAWAII HEALTH STORY

We started spending our vacations in Hawaii in our early 40's and enjoyed swimming, snorkeling, walking on the beach, and relaxing in the warm, sunny climate. Every year the stress in our lives increased and so did our waistlines. It was easy for us to ignore the worsening state of our bodies until our winter pilgrimage to Hawaii. Then, when squeezing into our bathing suits, we were confronted with how obese and out of shape we had become. Walking on the beach was more of a struggle every year and even getting out of the ocean after snorkeling was more difficult. Every year, after a week of relaxing in the Hawaiian sunshine, eating fish and fresh vegetables, and getting daily exercise, we always felt much better. And every year as we boarded the plane back to the mainland, we promised ourselves we would eat better and exercise more.

While living in Northern California, we tried everything to lose weight and feel better. We joined Weight Watchers, counted calories, and walked miles a day, but any weight loss was always short lived. We tried to find fresh fish and Hawaii grown fruits and vegetables to improve our diet but we could never find a consistent source. We sold our house and moved to another neighborhood in hopes of getting out of our rut. The change in location and residence did not help. The winters were still dark and cold, and food never satisfied us. We were always tired and stressed. Nothing we did changed our cycle of getting fatter, less fit, and feeling worse every year.

Everything we read about weight loss insisted that it was just simple arithmetic to eat less calories and exercise more. The only time the math worked for us was when were on vacation in Hawaii. Not only did we lose fat, walk faster, and feel more coordinated, we could not believe how much better we felt in Hawaii. Our trips to Hawaii became more frequent and we extended them longer. The more time we spent in Hawaii, the better we felt. Unfortunately, our happy, energetic feeling would fade away only a few weeks after returning to the mainland. Having a high-paid job and money in savings did not slow down the decline in our health. A fun-filled, active future for us seemed less and less likely as our mental and physical health declined every year.

At 50 we suddenly found ourselves unemployed and we resolved to take drastic action to make a real difference in our health and change our future. Since visiting Hawaii always made us feel better, we decided to spend a year in Hawaii to see if the weight loss and health improvements we experienced on vacations would be even greater if we lived there. We packed our belongings into a container and transported our cars to Hilo, a town with the lowest prices on rentals in Hawaii at the time.

We arrived in Hilo in November 2007 obese and exhausted. Almost immediately we started to feel better and have more energy in the warm climate. We started walking every day in Liliuokalani Gardens on Hilo Bay where the scenery is so uplifting it helped us ignore our out of shape bodies.

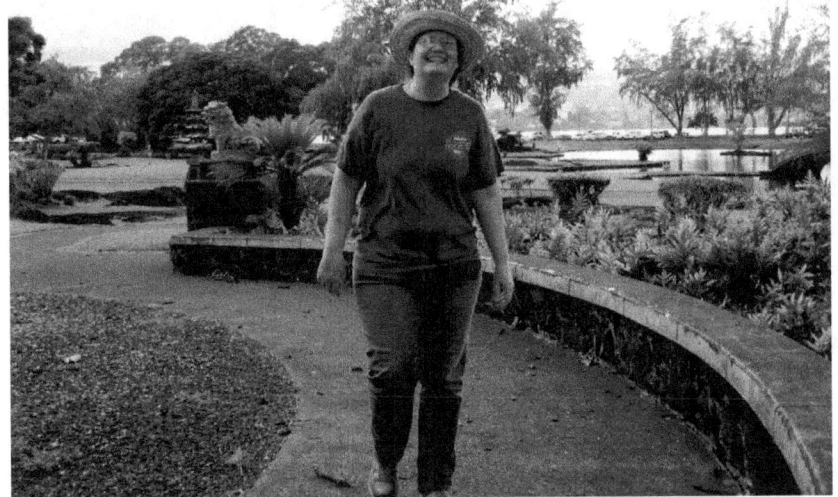

Chris exercising after arriving in Hawaii

Every morning was like awakening to a dream come true on the perfect summer day. The sun, the warmth, and a life without long commutes, stressful days, or trying to find healthy foods felt magical to us. Hilo has several Farmer's Markets with locally grown fruits and vegetables and a fish market selling the daily catch. Local grocery stores also sell island grown produce and Hawaii raised grass-fed beef.

We had a constant source of fresh, delicious, and nutritious food.

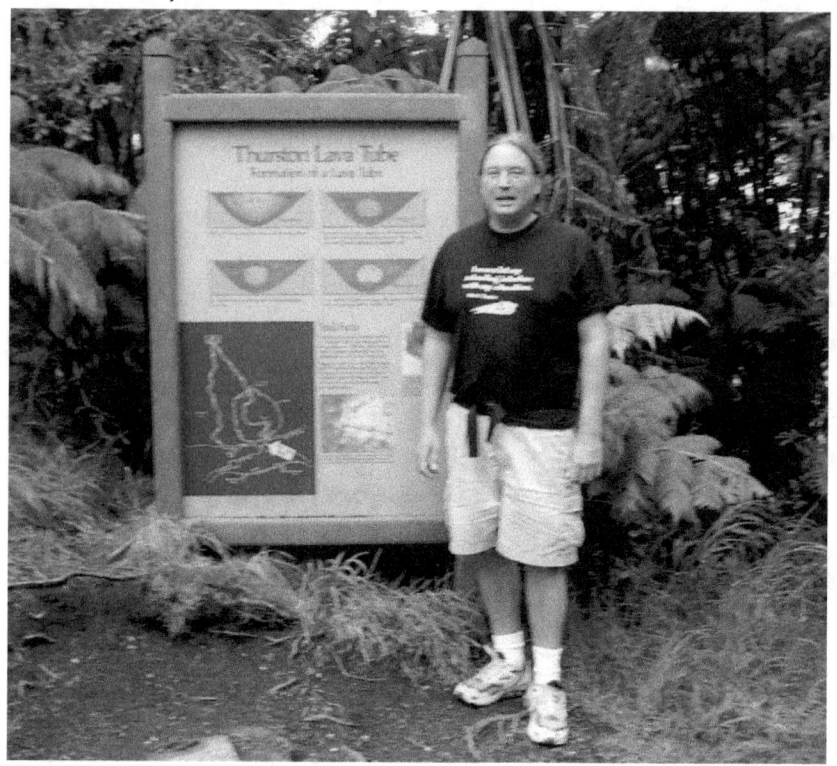

Tyler in Volcano after arriving in Hawaii

After getting settled into Hilo, we joined a water aerobics class, one of the few exercises we could do at the time. Many of the women in the group were in their 80's and 90's and we marveled at their level of fitness and boundless energy. In Hilo we met many energetic seniors, *kupuna* in Hawaiian, 20 to 40 years older than we were who made us feel old and decrepit. We wondered if living in Hawaii was the reason they had such remarkable health and longevity. If so, we wanted to have whatever they had too.

We met in high school in Indonesia and so we knew what it was like to live with rain, mold, and bugs in the tropics. We felt comfortable in Hilo's Asian and island culture. We have met many people who moved to Hawaii Island from the mainland and left within a year or two because they did not like the culture or living in the tropical climate. We have also met people who moved to Hawaii to enjoy the last months of their life after being diagnosed with terminal conditions and to their surprise they improved and had active and happy lives.

Our health started to improve during our first year in Hilo, however, it took us longer than we expected to decompress and slow down. We focused on familiarizing ourselves with the island, learning how to cook local foods, and catching up on 10 years of sleep deprivation. Our initial goals were to eat healthy foods, exercise regularly, and get under a Body Mass Index (BMI) of 30 so we were not obese. Our expenses for rent and food were much lower than in Northern California so our plan was to make our savings last as long as possible until we figured out what to do next. We continued to cut our spending dramatically and replaced our expensive medical insurance with Kaiser in Hawaii.

When our first year in Hawaii came to an end, we had made great progress, but we were still far from achieving our ultimate goal of having healthy weights, being fit, and feeling energetic. We knew we needed much more time in Hawaii. During our second year we came to the conclusion that returning to our stressful life on the mainland was unthinkable. We embarked on a plan to become writers, which gave us the time to exercise, shop for the healthiest foods, and cook.

As we lost weight and increased our daily exercise, we started having new health issues. The worst were Tyler's frequent and painful gout attacks. Gout is caused by high levels of uric acid in the blood that form crystals, usually in or near joints. Feet and hands are the most common places that the crystals form. In Tyler's case, they settled next to his big toe making walking nearly impossible. The long thin crystals act like needles and cut into the tissue and bone so that even touching the spot can cause intense pain. Since uric acid is not very soluble in water, it is hard to get the crystals to dissolve. We began the long process of removing foods, many that we had previously thought to be healthy, in hopes of decreasing his levels of uric acid.

We learned that canola oil (Canada oil low acid), which is touted as a healthy oil, was a genetically engineered version of rapeseed and historically considered inedible by humans due to its high erucic acid content. We also learned that fructose, which Tyler was getting a lot of from all the delicious Hawaiian fruits he ate every day, causes a rise in uric acid levels which increases the risk of gout attacks. We cut canola oil, fruit, syrup, honey, agave, corn, and all sugary foods from our diet.

Gout is common in Hilo, so everyone had a lot of sympathy for Tyler and they all shared their home remedies. Tyler tried many of them including drinking concentrated cherry juice, vinegar with the "mother", and topical treatments of aloe. The water on Hawaii Island has high levels of calcium leached from the lava. There are claims that calcium in drinking water can cause gout attacks because the high mineral content makes it harder to dissolve and remove uric acid from the body. We started drinking basic bottled water to help dissolve and flush out the uric acid. Maintaining an alkaline state helps deal with gout. Tyler also started taking malic acid which helps dissolve uric acid.

After two years in Hilo, we wanted to live somewhere on the island with more sun and snorkeling spots, so we moved to

Kona. Fortunately, rental prices had fallen in Kona since we arrived on the island and we were able to find a great condo on Alii Drive for less than our rental in Hilo. The condo complex was close to the beach and filled with fitness buffs. Year round residents in Kona were constantly biking, running, walking, swimming, and working out. We noticed people having remarkable improvement in their health after moving to Kona from the mainland. One man, we saw regularly shuffling along the road with a walker, was no longer using his walker within a year. The combination of sunny days and the fitness culture in Kona resulted in our having more energy to write, increasing our exercise, and making substantial progress on our weight loss.

Kona has many part-time residents who stay during the winter. We watched many of them lose weight and have incredible improvements in their health while they were in Kona, but when they returned a year later from the mainland some had lost all the progress they had made. We also met retirees in Kona who were fit and suddenly gained weight. Their setbacks worried us.

In our case, we were delighted to have made such great progress on our weight loss and fitness in Kona. We had achieved it through a strict, low calorie diet and lots of exercise. Suddenly, our progress stopped. We struggled with hunger, injuries from exercise, and Tyler's gout attacks returned. We urgently wanted to understand why the health benefits we had gotten in Kona had not lasted.

Through research and experimentation, we learned that it was not one thing but many things that were needed to have excellent health and maintain a healthy weight. Although Hawaii has everything we need for incredible health and vitality, it requires the right diet and amount of exercise for us to maintain it. This book shares what we learned during our seven years of getting healthy in Hawaii. We wish we had known this information years ago so we could have had more energy and better health in our 40's.

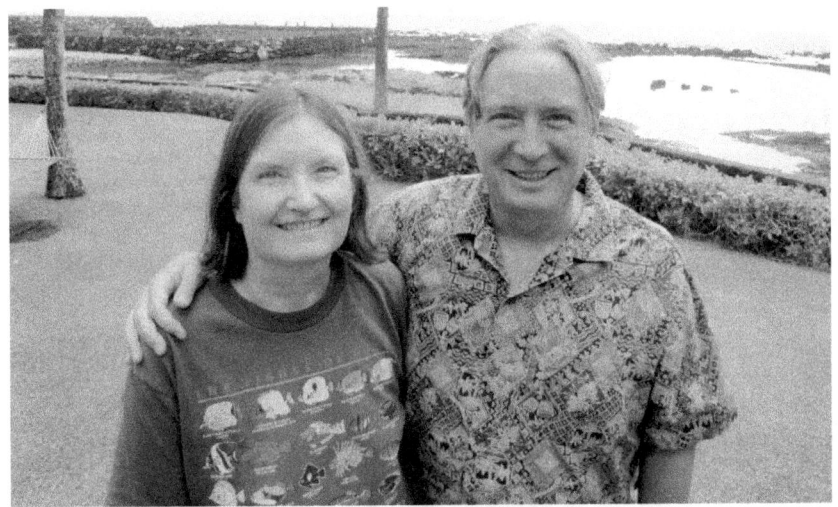

Feeling fantastic in Hawaii

Surprisingly, much of the information we learned that improved our health has been known for over a hundred years, but forgotten when antibiotics were discovered in the 1940's. Other research has only recently been published and some is still in the process of debate and further study. Although it took us a long time to find our recipe for health and vitality, we are thrilled with the results we achieved in Hawaii and excited about our future.

Chapter Two
INCREDIBLE SUNLIGHT IN HAWAII

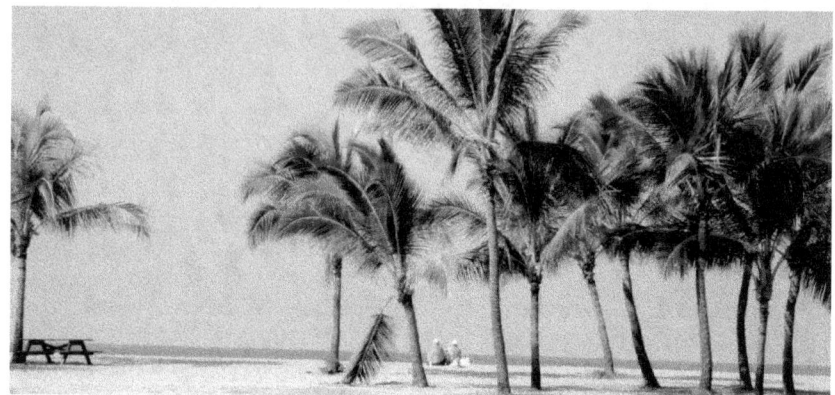

Sunbathing in Hawaii

The biggest attraction of Hawaii for us was the bright sunlight and warmth. When we arrived in Hawaii on our winter vacations, we would rush through the airport terminal to get into the sun as soon as possible. After months of overcast skies and rain on the mainland, the Hawaiian sunshine uplifted our spirits and the warmth caused our aches and pains to subside.

Is there more sunlight in Hawaii?

Hawaii is the southernmost and only place in the United States that is south of the Tropic of Cancer. It gets more direct sunlight than anywhere else in the nation. We thought after moving to Hawaii our attraction to the sunlight and its energizing effect would wear off. It did not. Having bright sunlight almost every day of the year is still a thrill to us and it makes every day feel like a vacation in Hawaii. It doesn't surprise us that studies have shown that sunlight and its visible and ultraviolet components dramatically improve health and happiness.

We remember the sunlight being brighter when we were kids. Sunlight has been dimming across the world for the past 50 years. Dr. Gerry Stanhill, an English scientist working in Israel, found a 22% drop in the sunlight in Israel since the 1950's.[1] He searched records from all around the world and found a drop in sunlight almost everywhere he looked. Sunlight decreased by 10% over the USA, nearly 30% in parts of eastern Europe, and 16% in parts of the British Isles. The global dimming is caused by pollution which reflects the sunlight back into space and keeps it from reaching the ground.

Polluted clouds are also reflective and block the sun's rays. Hawaii's remote location thousands of miles from any continent has protected it from much of the pollution being created in Asia and America.

Can sunlight improve your health?

Numerous studies have shown that sunlight improves health and prevents disease. In 2013 Han van der Rhee published a review of all the research on sunlight and cancer.[2] His conclusion was that constant sun exposure, and not occasional exposure, is associated with a reduced risk of colorectal cancer, breast cancer, prostate cancer, and non-Hodgkin's lymphoma.

Sunlight has ultraviolet components which are not visible but cause your skin to tan or burn. The ultraviolet wavelengths are classified as UVA, UVB and UVC, though most of the UVC never makes it through the atmosphere. When your skin gets UVB light, it turns a cholesterol-type compound into an initial form of inert vitamin D which becomes active vitamin D after several more processes in the body. During the winter in the northern latitudes, UVB light is so weak that exposed skin cannot start the first step in making vitamin D.[3]

So many health benefits have been tied to vitamin D that it has become a barometer of overall health. The primary health benefit of vitamin D is to help absorb calcium needed for bone health. However, people with low levels of vitamin D are more likely to die of cancer or heart disease or have other severe illnesses.[4]

Regular exposure to sunlight reduces the risk of getting rheumatoid arthritis. A study published in the *Annals of the Rheumatic Diseases* showed that participants with the most sunlight exposure were 21% less likely to get rheumatoid arthritis than those with the least exposure.[5] This research agrees with other studies that linked where people live and their risk of rheumatoid arthritis as well as other autoimmune diseases including type 1 diabetes, inflammatory bowel disease, and multiple sclerosis.[6]

After a week or more in Hawaii, people marvel as their aches and joint pains begin to subside. Visitors to Hawaii from the northern latitudes blissfully sunbathe in 75 degree winter days that we find a bit chilly. They excitedly show us movement in their previously immobile joints and point to places that used to hurt. Daily exposure to UVB from sunbathing most likely reduces their swelling.

Dr. Evropi Theodoratou at the University of Edinburgh and her team showed evidence that high levels of vitamin D lowers the risk for a long list of diseases including: colorectal cancer, non-vertebral fractures, cardiovascular disease, hypertension, stroke, depression, type 2 diabetes, reduced levels of balance sway, and chronic kidney disease.[7] In another study, Dr. Oscar H. Franco, a professor of preventive medicine in the Netherlands, showed adults with lower levels of vitamin D in their systems had a 35% increased risk of death from heart disease, 14% greater likelihood of death from cancer, and a greater risk of death overall.[8] Dr. Franco and his colleagues calculated that roughly 13% of all deaths in the United States and 9% in Europe could be attributed to low levels of vitamin D.

Some people are still short of vitamin D even with plenty of exposure to sunlight because the liver and the kidneys are needed to convert inert vitamin D to the active form of the vitamin. Vitamin D may not be converted if a person has liver or kidney problems, is taking medication that blocks the creation of cholesterol, or cannot absorb fat in the intestines. Obese people need twice as much vitamin D and are about 50% less efficient at utilizing UVB light compared to normal-weight people. The inert vitamin D remains in the fat and cannot be used by obese people. As we age, our skin absorbs less vitamin D from sunlight, so more sunlight is needed. Vitamin D studies have not shown that taking vitamin D pills are the same as getting vitamin D from sunlight.[9] Vitamin

D is in only a few foods, the primary source being fish, which are plentiful in Hawaii.

Can sunlight help you lose weight?

The brightness and amount of sunlight has been shown to help maintain a healthy weight. Dr. Kathryn Reid at Northwestern University's Feinberg School of Medicine in Chicago measured the light exposure of 54 volunteers and found that their Body Mass Index (BMI) was related to the brightness and amount of time they were exposed to light.[10] According to her research, the light intensity needs to be at least 500 Lux, and it is best to get the exposure early in the day. For every hour that light exposure was delayed, the study found that BMI's rose by 1.28 points.

After reading about the importance of brightness for the health benefits of sunlight we ordered a digital light meter to see how much light we get inside our home and on our daily walks. We measured the Lux during our early morning walks at 6:30AM. The sun was just on the horizon so were surprised to see the light readings already ranging from 800 to 3000 Lux. Later in the morning, sitting on our couch next to the open windows, the readings ranged from 500 to 600 Lux. At noon, on a cloudless day with the sunlight directly overhead, we measured over 140,000 Lux. These readings were taken during the summer when the sun is at its maximum. Even so, we are sure we get plenty of sunlight every day in Hawaii.

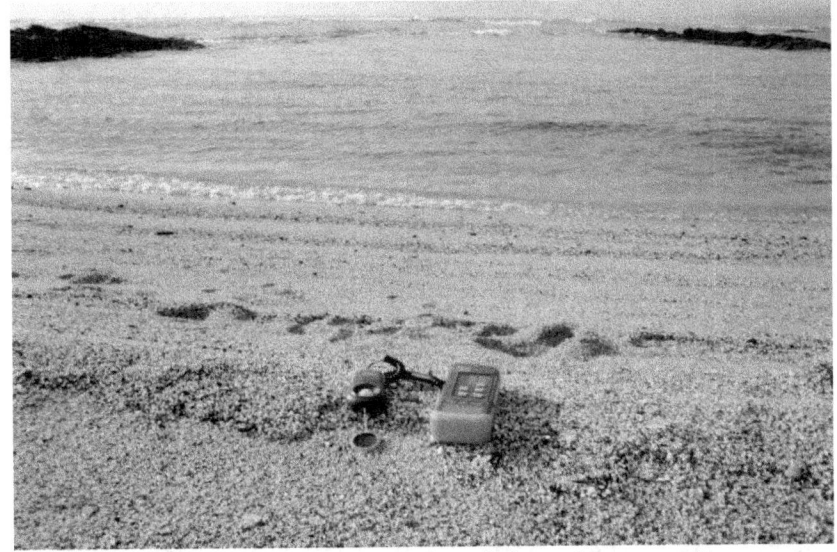

Measuring sunlight with a Luxmeter

When we lived in Northern California we created a "Hawaii Room" with a floor heater, full spectrum light bulbs, and calming Hawaiian music. Although it was nice to spend time in the room, it did not bring back the same level of happiness and energy we felt in Hawaii. In retrospect, the light source was clearly not bright enough to replicate 140,000 Lux and probably did not even meet the minimum 500 Lux found in the Feinberg School of Medicine study.

There are numerous ways exposure to sunlight helps with weight loss. Vitamin D, created by exposure to sunlight, helps regulate blood sugar levels, digest food, make fat cells more metabolically active, and rid the body of toxic wastes. It also increases the brain hormone leptin which makes you feel full. Overweight and obese people are usually deficient in vitamin D because the vitamin is locked inside their fat cells and cannot be used by the body. Nearly 3 of every 4 adolescent and adult Americans are deficient in vitamin D[11], which happens to be the same percentage of people who are overweight and obese.

Can sunlight increase your happiness?

One of our favorite components of sunlight is blue light. The eye is very sensitive to the blue color, which is more prevalent in the morning and a delight on walks along Hawaii's turquoise bays. Researchers at the University of Greenwich found that blue light makes people happier, more alert, and more productive.[12,13] Compared to the other light spectrums, blue light declines the most in the winter. However because of its southern latitude, Hawaii, has no loss of the blue spectrum light in the winter.

Recent research at Harvard Medical School has shown that constant exposure to ultraviolet light raises the levels of beta-endorphin, a natural opiate, in mice.[14] Previous studies found that giving an opioid blocker produces withdrawal-like symptoms in people who frequently suntan.[15]

The longer days and intense sunshine in Hawaii may account for the residents' lower BMIs, longer life spans, and greater happiness when compared to residents on the mainland. Having intense sunlight and blue spectrum light all year long solves part of the mystery of why when we are in Hawaii we feel so energetic, active, and happy.

References:
1. G. Stanhill and S. Moreshet, "Global radiation climate changes in Israel," *Climatic Change*, 22 (1992): 121-138.
2. Han van der Rhee, Jan Willem Coebergh, and Esther de Vries, "Is prevention of cancer by sun exposure more than just the effect of vitamin D? A systematic review of epidemiological studies," *European Journal of Cancer* 49, no. 6 (2013): 1422–1436.
3. M. Wacker and M. F. Holick, "Vitamin D – effects on skeletal and extraskeletal health and the need for supplementation," *Nutrients* 5, no. 1 (2013): 111–148.
4. M. F. Holick and T. C. Chen, "Vitamin D deficiency: a worldwide problem with health consequences," *American Journal of Clinical Nutrition* 87, no. 4 (2008): 1080S-6S.
5. E. V. Arkema and others, "Exposure to ultraviolet-B and risk of developing rheumatoid arthritis among women in the Nurses' Health Study," *Annals of Rheumatic Diseases*, 72, no 4 (2013): 506-11.

6. C. F. Garland and others, "The Role of vitamin D in cancer prevention," *American Journal of Public Health* 96, no 2 (2006): 252-261.

7. Evropi Theodoratou and others, "Vitamin D and multiple health outcomes: umbrella review of systematic reviews and meta-analyses of observational studies and randomized trials," *BMJ*, 348 (April 2014): g2035.

8. Rajiv Chowdhury, Oscar H. Franco and others, "Vitamin D and risk of cause specific death: systematic review and meta-analysis of observational cohort and randomised intervention studies," *BMJ*, 348 (2014): g1903.

9. Karin Amrein and others, "Effect of High-Dose Vitamin D_3 on Hospital Length of Stay in Critically Ill Patients With Vitamin D Deficiency: The VITdAL-ICU Randomized Clinical Trial," *JAMA* 312, no 15 (2014): 1520-1530.

10. K.J. Reid and others, "Timing and Intensity of Light Correlate with Body Weight in Adults," *PLoS ONE* 9, no 4 (2014): e92251.

11. Adit A. Ginde, Mark C. Liu, and Carlos A. Camargo Jr., "Demographic differences and trends of vitamin D insufficiency in the US Population, 1988-2004," *Archive of Internal Medicine* 169, no 6 (2009): 626-632.

12. A. U. Viola and others, "Blue-enriched white light in the workplace improves self-reported alertness, performance and sleep quality," *Scandinavian Journal of Work, Environment & Health,* 34, no 4 (2008): 297-306.

13. S. Lehrl and others, "Blue light improves cognitive performance," *Journal of Neural Transmission* 114 no. 4 (2007): 457-460

14. Sue McGreevey, "Addicted to the Sun: Research in mice connects UV light to opiate-like effects," *Harvard Medical School News* (June 19,

2014) website:
http://hms.harvard.edu/news/addicted-sun-6-19-14
last accessed 12/1/2014.
15. B. V. Nolan and others, "Tanning as an addictive behavior: a literature review," *Photodermatology Photoimmunology Photomedicine Journal* 25, no 1 (2009):12-19.

Chapter Three
ENERGIZING IODINE IN HAWAII'S OCEAN

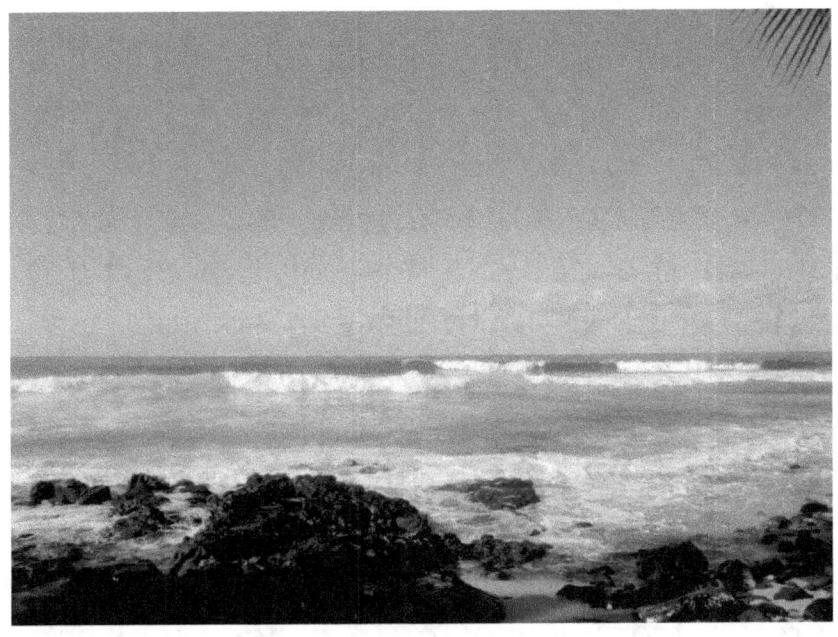

We have always loved the ocean. In college we would drive an hour to the Oregon coast even during the cold winters, park our car facing the crashing waves, and study. Something about the ocean invigorates us and we feel better being near it. Now that we live in Hawaii, we walk along the coastline every evening and find a place to sit and let the salty mist envelope us until sunset. Our research into the benefits of iodine explains why the ocean makes us feel so good.

Is there a shortage of iodine in our diet?

Iodine is a vital nutrient needed by the thyroid gland in your neck to control the body's metabolism and by every cell and gland in the body. Most of the earth's iodine is stored in the ocean so you can get it by eating fish and sea vegetables and produce grown in soil near the ocean. A minimum amount of iodine was added to table salt to prevent mental retardation in babies and keep the thyroid from swelling, called goiter. However, anyone who lives more than 100 miles from the coast is at risk of being iodine deficient and it may be worse if you don't eat seafood and you avoid iodized salt.[1]

Some of the many symptoms of low functioning thyroid (hypothyroidism) caused by lack of iodine include weight gain, cold hands and feet, hair loss, low energy, muscle weakness, constipation, throat pain, muscle cramps, depression, dry skin, poor memory, slow heartbeat, and cysts. [2]   This sounds a lot like us before we moved to Hawaii.

Dr. David Brownstein's book, *Iodine: Why you need it; Why you can't live without it,* was a big "ah ha!" for us. It explained why we have always been drawn to the ocean and feel so invigorated by being close to it. It may even explain some of the miraculous health improvements we have seen in people after they move to Hawaii and spend every day near the ocean breathing in the ocean spray.

The lack of iodine in American's diet has worsened in recent decades because of changes to food and more exposure to iodine-blocking chemicals.   Iodine is chemically similar to the other halogen elements fluorine, chlorine, and bromine. Exposure to compounds with fluorine, chlorine, and bromine can block iodine absorption and disrupt the thyroid's functioning.

In the 1970's, potassium bromate replaced potassium iodide in wheat flour as a bread conditioner. Most of the rest of world banned the additive when it was shown to cause thyroid and kidney cancer in rats and mice.[3] In the United States most processed bread and baked foods have residues of bromine. We are exposed to bromine in many other products as well. Bromated vegetable oil is used as an emulsifier in many citrus flavored sodas. Bromine is added to clothing, bedding, car interiors, and couches as a flame retardant. Bromine is used to treat water in swimming pools and hot tubs and is an ingredient in pesticides. Bromine compounds are also in many common medicines including painkillers, sedatives, and antihistamines.

In addition to bromine, fluorine and chlorine compounds are everywhere in our environment. Fluoride is in drinking water, toothpaste, mouthwash, and chewing gum. Percholate, a compound of chlorine and oxygen, has been shown to disrupt the thyroid. It is a common contaminate in drinking water and used in fireworks, airbags, and rocket fuel. Exposure to these chemicals in the environment causes them to build up in the body and increases the likelihood of being iodine deficient.

Some natural substances, called goitirogens, also block iodine absorption into the body. Vegetables such as cabbage, brussels sprouts, cauliflower, broccoli, turnips, kale, collard greens, and radishes as well as legumes such as soybeans, peas, and lentils contain goitirogens. Fortunately most goitirogens are destroyed by the heat when they are cooked.[1]

Soy goitirogens, however, are not destroyed by heat. Soy products are said to be in over 60% of the foods in grocery stores added as flour, texturized vegetable protein, and vegetable oil. Only fermentation destroys the anti-thyroid substances in soy which is how it is eaten in Asia in the form of miso, tempeh, natto, and soy sauce.[1] While living on the mainland, we ate a lot of soy products and never realized that they were lowering our metabolism and may have been partly responsible for our low energy and feeling cold.

We had no idea that our food, drinks, clothes, furniture, and so many of the products in our environment increased our risk of being iodine deficient.

Can iodine improve your health?

In 1829, a French physician Jean Lugol discovered that a solution of potassium iodide and iodine treated infections and numerous other ailments. "Lugol's Solution" was a major breakthrough in the medical world and was widely prescribed by physicians before being replaced by antibotics.[2]

The use of iodine to treat breast cancer dates back to 1896.[2] It has been known for five decades that low iodine levels result in cysts and ultimately cancer in the breasts, ovaries, uterus, and prostate where iodine is concentrated. Dr. Stadel suggested in 1976 that there were lower rates of cancers of the prostate, uterus, ovary and breast in populations that have diets with high iodine content.[5]

An adult with enough iodine has about 15 to 20 mg of iodine concentrated in the thyroid gland. However, this accounts for only about 30% of the body's iodine. The rest is found in breast tissue, eyes, gastrointestinal tract, cervix, salivary glands, bones, and body fluids. Iodine has been shown to have an antioxidant function in mammary tissues, however, the function of iodine in other parts of the body is still unknown. [7]

Without sufficient iodine, the thyroid cannot make enough hormones to stimulate the mitochondria to produce energy (ATP). The lack of energy contributes to muscle soreness, fatigue, and brain fog.[2] Dr. Brownstein describes the benefits of taking 100 times the recommended dosage for iodine to protect against cancer. When plenty of iodine is available to the body, organs other than the thyroid have access to iodine. One of the benefits of iodine being available beyond the thyroid's requirements is that programmed cell death, called apoptosis, is restored.[2] Numerous diseases can result from apoptosis being interrupted or slowed in its task of killing billions of cells each day.

The Japanese consume at least 35 to 90 times the US recommended dosage of iodine (RDA of 150 mcg) from seaweed such as kombu and fish in their diet. Although their intake of iodine is far above the 1 mg "safety limit" of US standards, the Japanese have had no negative effects to their thyroids'. In fact, the Japanese have less hypothyroidism, goiter, breast cancer, ovarian cancer, and prostate cancer.[6,7]

In Hawaii, iodine in the ocean mist covers the grasslands and filters into the ground water. Locally grown vegetables and fruits are bathed in the mist and iodine-rich fish from the ocean are a major part of the diet. Spending time in Hawaii relieves muscle soreness and fatigue partly because of the iodine in the air, food, and water.

Can Iodine help you get off caffeine?

After learning about the dangers of all the chemicals we are exposed to that block iodine absorption, we started iodine supplements. Dr. Brownstein recommends adults take 12 to 50 mg a day.[2] We started taking 5 drops of 2% Lugol's Solution in a large glass of water every morning.

Taking iodine supplements can start a detox reaction as your body gets rid of the stored fluoride, bromide, perchlorate, and metals like mercury, lead, aluminum, and cadmium. The iodine breaks the toxins free which can bring on symptoms such as tiredness, irritability, diarrhea, nausea, and extra mucus.[2] In our case we felt tired and uncomfortable for about two weeks and then much better. People report that the symptoms can last longer depending on the accumulation of halogens and other chemicals in the body and if you continue to be exposed to the chemicals in your environment or food.[5]

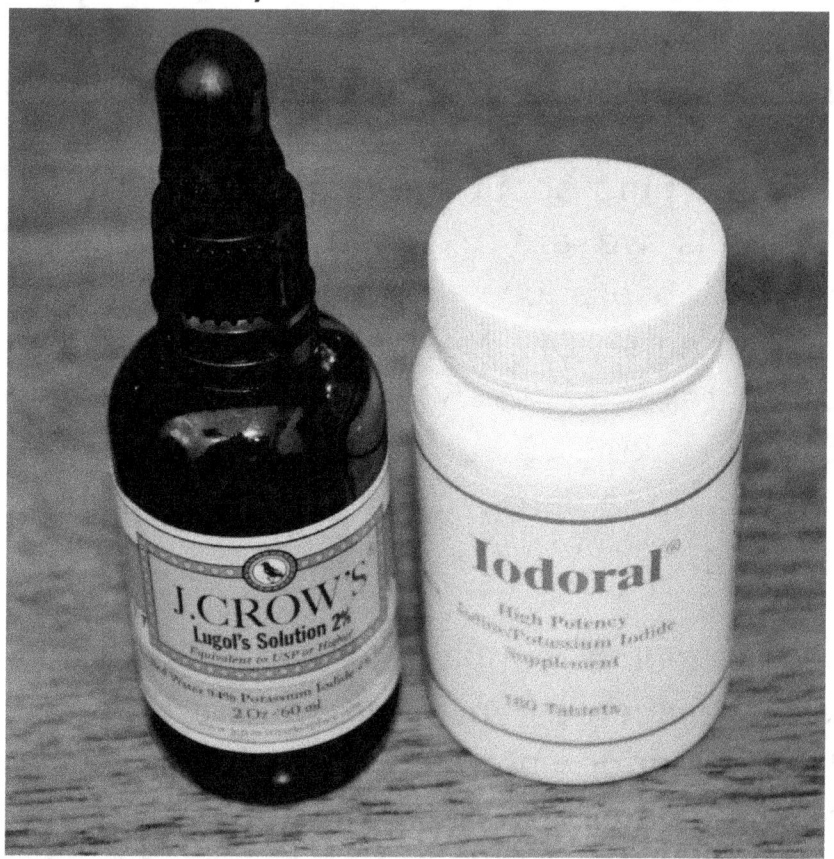

Lugol's Solution in drops and pill form

After getting past the initial detox phase, we suddenly had so much energy we were hyperactive. Ever since high school we have been heavy coffee drinkers needing two pots of coffee to get going in the morning and another large cup in the afternoon. After our iodine supplement in the morning, we noticed we drank less coffee. We cut out our afternoon coffee and slowly reduced the number of cups we drank in the morning. After two months, coffee no longer tasted good to us and we stopped drinking it.

We knew that too much caffeine can cause anxiety, sleep problems, spasms, dehydration, and stomach upset, but we did not know that just 200 mg of caffeine increases the cortisol levels in the blood by 30% within an hour.[8] Cortisol reduces metabolism, increases belly fat, and causes the body to breakdown muscle tissue. Cortisol also reduces leptin, the hormone that regulates hunger, so you feel hungry no matter how much food you have eaten.

Caffeine causes the blood vessels to be constricted; one study showed that just 250 mg of caffeine reduced blood flow to the brain by 30%.[9] This is scary since caffeine also increases blood pressure, a combination that increases the risk of stroke. Without caffeine the blood flow increases to the brain and can cause headaches. On the upside the additional blood and oxygen to the brain increases concentration and memory, but it also helped us to remember how much we loved our morning coffee. Taking painkillers for the headache from lack of caffeine is not helpful as many painkillers contain caffeine.

We have more energy and better concentration now from taking iodine supplements. We wake up earlier and sleep better. We spend less time being upset, worrying, and being hungry. Even more surprising has been the bottle of wine we drank every night to help us fall asleep is no longer needed. We no longer need to counter the effects of caffeine in the evening with alcohol.

The iodine in the ocean mist that surrounds the Hawaiian Islands is part of the mystery of why people in Hawaii have more energy, better health, and live longer.

References:
1. Bruce Fife, *The Coconut Ketogenic Die*t (Colorado Springs: Piccadilly Books, 2014).
2. David Brownstein, *Iodine: Why you need it; Why you can't live without it,* 5th Edition, (Michigan: Medical Alternatives Press, 2014).
3. Y. Kurokawa and others, "Toxicity and carcinogenicity of potassium bromate – a new renal carcinogen," *Environmental Health Perspectives* 87(1990): 309-335.
4. B. V. Stadel, "Dietary iodine and risk of breast, endometrial, and ovarian cancer," *Lancet* 1, no. 7965 (1976): 890-1.
5. Lynne Farrow, *The Iodine Crisis: What you don't know about Iodine Can Wreck your Life* (New York: Devon Press, 2013).
6. Y. Fuse, "Smaller thyroid gland volume with high urinary iodine excretion in Japanese school children: normative reference values in an iodine-sufficient area and comparison with the WHO/ICCIDD reference," *Thyroid.* 17, no. 2 (2007): 145–155.
7. L. Patrick, "Iodine: deficiency and therapeutic considerations," *Alt Medical Review* 13, no. 2 (2008):116–127.
8. William R. Lovallo and others, "Stress-like adrenocorticotropin responses to caffeine in young healthy men" *Pharmacology Biochemistry and Behavior* 55, no. 3 (1996): 365-9.
9. Stephen Cherniske, *Caffeine Blues: Wake up to the Hidden Dangers of America's #1 Drug* (New York: Warner Books, 1998).

Chapter Four
AMAZING COCONUT OIL

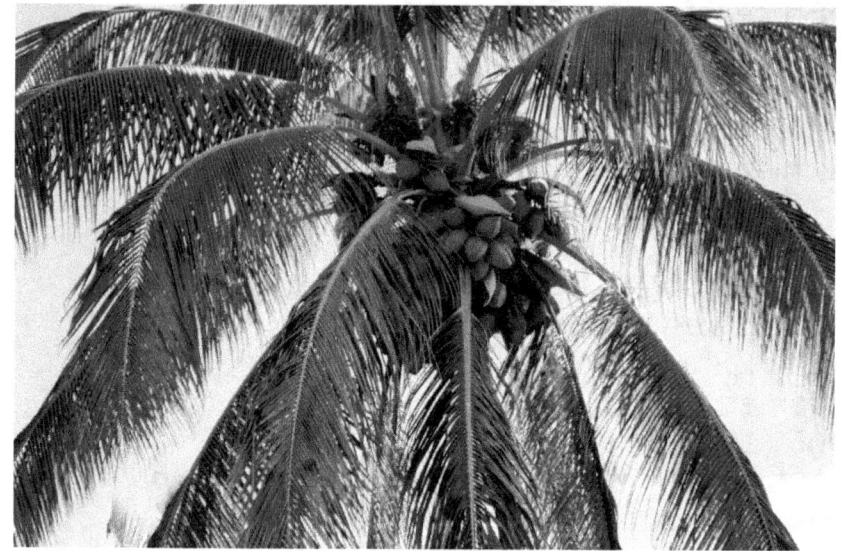

Hawaii coconut tree

We have always wanted to live in Hawaii to be back in a tropical climate. We met in Jakarta, Indonesia while attending high school and fell in love with its intense sunlight and continuous summer climate. We remember the feeling of being healthy and happy in Indonesia's tropical climate. Our vacations to Hawaii convinced us that moving to the sunny islands would give us the energy and health we enjoyed in high school. What we didn't realize while living in Indonesia was that our diet of seafood and coconut oil was also responsible for our health, energy, and weight loss. Coconut and palm seed oils from the tropics have healthy properties that are not found in vegetable oils.

Is coconut oil good for you?

Coconut oil was widely used in the United States until the 1950's for baking and frying and in processed foods like crackers and cookies. A prominent diet researcher, Dr. Ancel Keys, proposed the theory that saturated fats in American's diet was causing an increase in heart disease. A campaign against saturated fats claimed that butter, eggs and coconut oil were unhealthy. Although there was no proof that dietary fat had anything to do with heart disease, low-fat diets were recommended by the American Heart Association and Dr. Keys made the cover of Time Magazine in 1961.[1,2]

Restaurants and food companies replaced coconut oil and animal fats with polyunsaturated "vegetable oils" processed from corn, soy beans, cotton seeds, and rape seeds. Vegetable oils are made up primarily of long-chain triglycerides (LCTs) which are easily broken down when exposed to heat, light, and oxygen and become toxic when they go rancid. Heat is normally used during the process of making vegetable oil, however, refined oils have been deodorized so you cannot tell that the oil is rancid. [1]

In the case of rape seed oil, rebranded as "Canola oil", the seeds are initially pressed and then washed for an hour in a chemical solvent to extract more oil. The seed cake remaining is used for animal feed. The oil is rinsed with sodium hydroxide and then cooled to separate out the wax which is used for vegetable shortening. Finally the oil is bleached to lighten the color and steam heated to remove the foul odor of the oil. [3]

In contrast, coconut oil is separated just by boiling the coconut meat in water or letting the juice squeezed from coconut meat sit in a container for 24 to 36 hours. Saturated fats, like coconut oil, are chemically more stable and resistant to oxidization and free-radical formation. Coconut oil can be exposed to light, oxygen, and heat without going rancid.[4]

The cold press processing of polyunsaturated vegetable oils lowers the amount of oxidization, however, the oil must be stored in dark glass and has a limited shelf life before becoming rancid. If heated for cooking, even cold pressed vegetable oils create unhealthy trans fatty acids.[1]

Although a diet with vegetable oils has been shown to lower cholesterol levels, new studies link vegetable oils to increased death rates from cardiovascular disease and coronary artery disease.[5] The saturated fats in meat, butter, and tropical oils were thought to be a problem because they increase low density lipoprotein (LDL) cholesterol, but there is no evidence to support the claim that saturated fats increase coronary risk.[6] In fact, studies have shown that eating a lot of saturated fats, up to 50% of total daily calories, has little to no effect on total cholesterol or LDL.[1] These studies convinced us to remove all vegetable oils from our diet and replace them with coconut oil.

In an article published by the Mayo Clinic, Dr. Ravnskov and others found that some studies condemning saturated fats had classified processed foods with carbohydrates as "saturated fats" and that the UK government and National Institute of Clinical Excellence list biscuits, cakes, pastries and savory snacks as "saturated fats". [7]

Studies published in the *Philippine Journal of Internal Medicine* and the *American Journal of Clinical Nutrition* of coconut consuming people in Polynesia and elsewhere in the tropics have shown that eating coconut oil does not lead to high cholesterol in the blood or to an increase in coronary heart disease or death.[8,9]

It turns out that LDL has different shapes and sizes and medical research has shown that the big "fluffy LDL" particles from saturated fats like coconut oil and cholesterol are not the problem. It is the small, dense LDL particles that readily oxidize and can slip through the walls of the arteries that cause the formation of problem plaque. The small, dense LDL particles responsible for the risk factors related to heart attacks and strokes are caused by eating sugar and high carbohydrate diets.[10] Studies have shown that saturated fats actually lower the concentration of small, dense LDL and raise the concentration of the large, fluffy LDL.[11]

This goes against everything we have been told by the medical profession and in the news. All of our attempts to lose weight on low-fat diets, mostly consisting of carbohydrates, increased our risk of heart attack and stroke. It is ironic that all the years we denied ourselves fat to improve our health, we were actually harming our health.

Can coconut oil help you lose weight?

Studies have reported that adding coconut oil to your diet is an effective way to lose weight, body fat, and reduce waist size.[12] Tropical oils, like coconut oil, are digested differently than other fats and are quickly converted to energy. Coconut oil increases your metabolism and reduces your appetite.

Coconut oil is rapidly digested without the need for bile or pancreatic enzymes. It is carried by the portal vein directly to the liver where it is immediately converted to energy. The speed of metabolism of coconut oil by the body is similar to the metabolism of sugar and carbohydrates, except that medium chain triglycerides (MCTs) from coconut oil are not deposited as fat.[1] This unique property of coconut oil explains why we lost weight and were so energetic living on Indonesian foods.

Animal fats and vegetable oils are mostly long-chain triglycerides (LCTs) which need bile from the liver and pancreatic enzymes to be digested. The digested fats are packaged into bundles with proteins called lipoproteins and circulated in the bloodstream to distribute them throughout the body. When the remaining lipoproteins arrive in the liver, they are either used to produce energy if needed or stored as fat.

In 1951 Dr Pennington determined that the body can burn unlimited amounts of fat, but is limited in the amount of carbohydrates it can burn.[13] According to Pennington, people are obese because the carbohydrates they eat are turning into fat even on strict low-calorie diets. Pennington's low-carbohydrate diet was called the "DuPont Diet" and published in 1950.

A low carbohydrate/high fat diet, or ketogenic diet, produces energy in the body from fat instead of glucose. If there is no glucose in the blood or stored as glycogen in the liver, then the liver converts fat to ketones for energy. No matter how many carbohydrates are eaten, the liver can only store about 2000 calories as glycogen; the rest is converted to fat. Although glycogen can be quickly converted to energy, once it is gone the muscles and brain stop functioning; we have seen this happen to Ironman athletes in Kona.

When the body is using fat, or ketones, for fuel, it can convert up to 40,000 calories a day, 20 times more than from glucogen. Ketones are created from fatty acids in the liver when glucose levels fall. Ketones are burned by the body differently and produce much less CO_2 than glycogen so you can exercise more before you are out of breath. There are other benefits to ketogenic energy including better efficiency of the muscles, like the heart.[1] After switching to a ketogenic diet, we finally made great progress on our weight loss and found it much easier to maintain. We also notice an increase in our energy and spend longer periods of time doing house cleaning and other chores before needing a rest.

A ketogenic diet with coconut oil gives us more energy as well as assisting in weight loss. A study in Italy showed an increase in metabolism of subjects after a meal that included just 2 tablespoons of coconut oil.[15] The normal weight subjects had an increase in their metabolism of 48% and the overweight subjects over 65%. The increase in metabolism from a meal with coconut oil has been shown to last up to 24 hours. Increasing our metabolic rate with coconut oil allows us to go hours between meals without being hungry.

In the tropical climate of Hawaii, coconut oil is always liquid at room temperature just like vegetable oil. Even in the tropics coconut oil does not need to be refrigerated and has a shelf life of up to two years because of its resistance to heat and oxidization. We use coconut oil exactly the same way as vegetable oil in our salads and dressings. We also use it to fry eggs and fish and for baking.

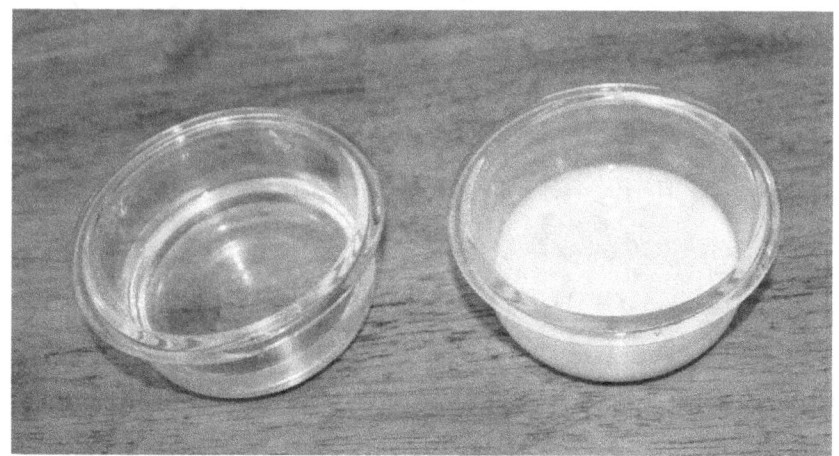

Coconut oil and creamed Coconut meat

We also eat coconut meat. We buy it ground up with the oil, which is called "creamed coconut", not to be confused with coconut cream. We mix the creamed coconut into sauces, stews, and use it for baking. It is amazing to us that a food as delicious as coconut also supports our weight loss and increases our energy.

Can coconut oil improve your health?

Coconut is more than a delicious and healthy food, it is medicine that kills many types of bacteria, viruses, protozoa, and parasites that antibiotics cannot kill. In contrast to antibiotics, it does not harm the helpful bacteria in our bodies. A study of Candida in Nigeria showed that coconut oil was able to treat fungal infections.[14]

It is able to do this because most bacteria, viruses, and protozoa (parasites) are covered with a thin "skin" of oil very similar to coconut oil's medium chain fatty acids which can combine with this "skin" oil and break it up so the body's white blood cells can destroy the pathogens.[4]

Lauric acid is the primary saturated fatty acid in coconut oil. It also contains myristic acid, capric acid, caprylic acid, and caproic acid which have antimicrobial properties that kill or slow down the growth of bacteria. Lauric acid is converted into monolaurin in the body, which has anti-viral, anti-microbial, anti-parasitic, and anti-fungal properties and helps the immune system. The compound monolaurin is a treatment for fungal infections, bacterial infections and fat-coated viruses. Breast milk is the only other natural source that contains such high concentration of lauric acid. Caprylic acid is a natural yeast fighting substance and kills Candida cells and other fungi.[4]

In addition to healthy oil, coconut has the vitamins C, B1, B2, B3, E, and Folate in the meat. It also has the minerals calcium, iron, copper, magnesium, manganese, phosphorus, potassium, sodium, zinc, and amino acids. Coconut oil from the tropics is less expensive than imported vegetable oil in Hawaii and it is commonly used in local, Polynesian, and Asian dishes. We not only eat the amazing and delicious coconut, we put the oil on our skin and hair for its curative properties.

Coconut oil is one of the reasons people in Hawaii are healthier and more energetic.

References

1. Bruce Fife, *The Coconut Ketogenic Diet* (Colorado Springs: Piccadilly Books, 2014).
2. John Tierney, "Diet and Fat: A Severe Case of Mistaken Consensus," *New York Times*, (October 2007) website:
http://www.nytimes.com/2007/10/09/science/09tier.html
last accessed on 12/1/2014.
3. How Its Made - Canola Oil, video website:
http://youtube.com/watch?v=omjWmLG0EAs
Last accessed on 12/1/2014.
4. Bruce Fife, *The Coconut Oil Miracle* (New York: Penguin Group, 2013).
5. Rajiv Chowdhury and others, "Association of Dietary, Circulating, and Supplement Fatty Acids With Coronary Risk: A Systematic Review and Meta-analysis," *Annals of Internal Medicine* 160, no. 6 (2014): 398-406.
6. Richard Bazinet and Michael W.A. Chu "Omega-6 polyunsaturated fatty acids: Is a broad cholesterol-lowering health claim appropriate?," *Canadian Medical Association Journal*, 186 (2013):434-439.
7. Uffe Ravnskov and others, "The questionable benefits of exchanging saturated fat with polyunsaturated fat," *Mayo Clinic Proceedings* 89, no. 4 (2014):451-3.
8. H. Kaunitz and C. S. Dayrit, "Coconut oil consumption and coronary heart disease," *Philippine Journal of Internal Medicine* 30 (1992):165-171.
9. I.A. Prior and others, "Cholesterol, coconuts, and diet on Polynesian atolls: a natural experiment: the Pukapuka and Tokelau island

studies,". *American Journal of Clinical Nutrition* 34, no. 8 (1981):1552-1561.

10. John Hopkins Medicine, "The New Blood Lipid Tests - Sizing Up LDL Cholesterol," *Health Alerts,* (June 13, 2008) website:
http://www.johnshopkinshealthalerts.com/reports/heart_health/1886-1.html
last accessed on 12/1/2014.

11. D. M. Dreon and others, "Change in dietary saturated fat intake is correlated with change in mass of large low-density-lipoprotein particles in men," *American Journal of Clinical Nutrition* 67, no. 5 (1998): 828-836.

12. H. Tsuji and others, "Dietary medium-chain triglycerols suppress accumulation of body fat in a double-blind, controlled trial in healthy men and women," *Journal of Nutrition* 131 (2001): 2853-2859.

13. Alfred Pennington, "The Use of Fat in a Weight-reducing diet," *Journal of the Medical Society of Delaware* (April 1951).

14. D. O. Ogbolu, "In vitro antimicrobial properties of coconut oil on Candida species in Ibadan, Nigeria," *Journal of Medicinal Food*, 10, no. 2 (2007):384-7.

15. L. Scalfi, A, Coltorti, and F. Contaldo, "Postprandial thermogenesis in lean and obese subjects after meals supplemented with medium-chain and long-chain triglycerides,". *American Journal of Clinical Nutrition* 53, no. 5 (1991):1130-3.

Chapter Five
LOCALLY GROWN FOODS IN HAWAII

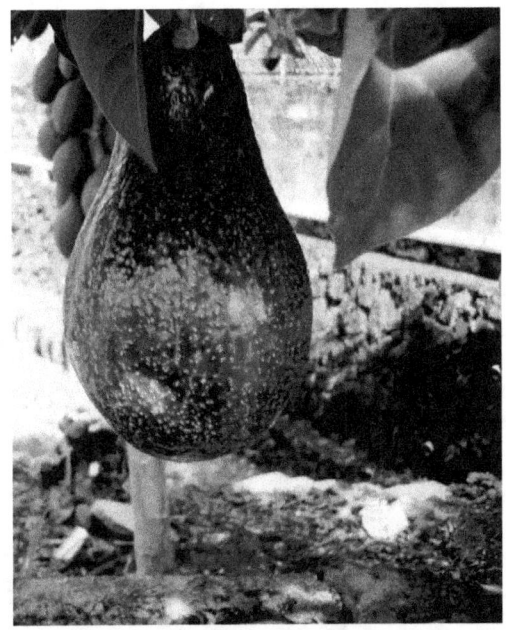

Hawaii Avocado tree

In Hawaii, the farms, cattle ranches, and ocean keep Farmer's Markets and local stores stocked with fresh vegetables, beef, pork, chicken, and fish. Having access to nutritious foods year round is one of the ways many people in Hawaii stay healthy and live long.

Does eating fish improve your health?

The ocean surrounding the Hawaiian Islands is teeming with fish that provide delicious meals with protein, vitamins, iodine, calcium, phosphorus, and selenium. More importantly, ocean fish are one of the few foods that provide essential omega-3 fatty acids to the body. Omega-3 fatty acids in fish have been found to prevent heart disease, reduce the risk of Alzheimer's disease, and prevent eye disease.[1,2,3,4] Some people are concerned about the contaminants found in fish, but other than for women of childbearing age, the magnitude of the health benefits from eating fish has been shown to exceed the potential risks.[6]

Clinical trials found that people who ate only 4 ounces of fatty fish, like tuna, each week reduced their risk of cardiovascular death by 36% compared with those who ate no fish at all. It is believed that the omega-3 fatty acids in fish are providing the protection.[1]

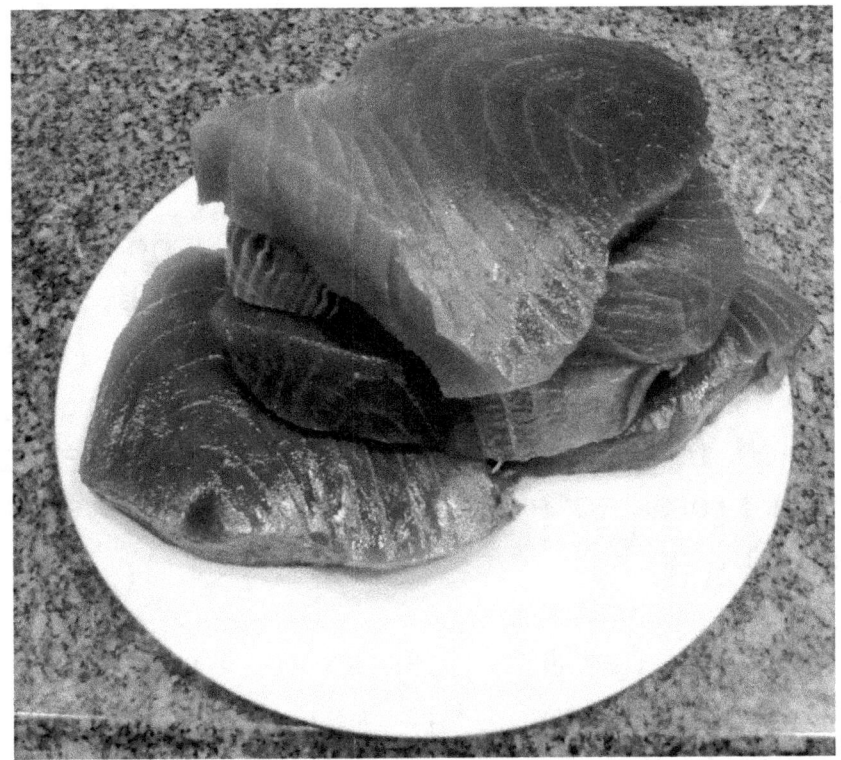

Hawaii Ahi (Tuna)

Docosahexaenoic acid (DHA) is an omega-3 fatty acid found throughout the body, but it is most concentrated in the brain. As we age, DHA levels decrease in the brain. Eating fish may help keep DHA levels higher in the brain and protect it from aging and dementia. The Framingham Heart Study followed 900 healthy men and women ranging in age from 55 to 88 years old for nine years.[2] Researchers found that the participants in the study who ate three servings of fish every week lowered their risk of developing dementia by 47% and lowered their risk of developing Alzheimer's disease by 39% compared with people who ate little or no fish.[3] Another recent study of 2,300 people in Finland aged 65 and older showed that participants who ate baked or broiled fish three or more times a week were protected from memory loss as well as from strokes.[4]

Eating fish has also been shown to protect the eyes because the retina is largely made of DHA. A study showed that just one portion of fish a week reduces the risk of age-related macular degeneration in the eye by 50%.[5]

Most Americans do not get enough omega-3's in their diet and some have none at all. Symptoms of an omega-3 deficiency in the diet include fatigue, poor memory, dry skin, heart problems, mood swings, depression, and poor circulation. Researchers have also linked cancer, diabetes, and other chronic diseases to low levels of omega-3.

Before moving to Hawaii, we rarely ate fish however, during our vacations to the islands we could never get enough of the local fish. The freshness and variety of fish in Hawaii make it more appealing to us. Every season different types of fish and marine life show up in Hawaiian waters and are available in grocery stores and from local fishermen. Hawaii has fatty fish such as Ahi (Tuna), Tombu (Albacore), Aku (Skipjack), Mahimahi (Dolphin fish), Opah (Moonfish), Ono (Wahoo), Onaga (Long-tail red snapper), and shellfish. Fish is in every grocery store and on every menu in Hawaii. Living in Hawaii has increased the amount of fish we eat.

Is grass-fed beef healthier?

Cattle are raised on the lush grasses that grow on the slopes of Hawaii's volcanoes. Grass grows year round in Hawaii, so ranchers do not have to store feed for the winter or move the cattle. The cattle are free to roam, antibiotics are not required, and hormones are not used.

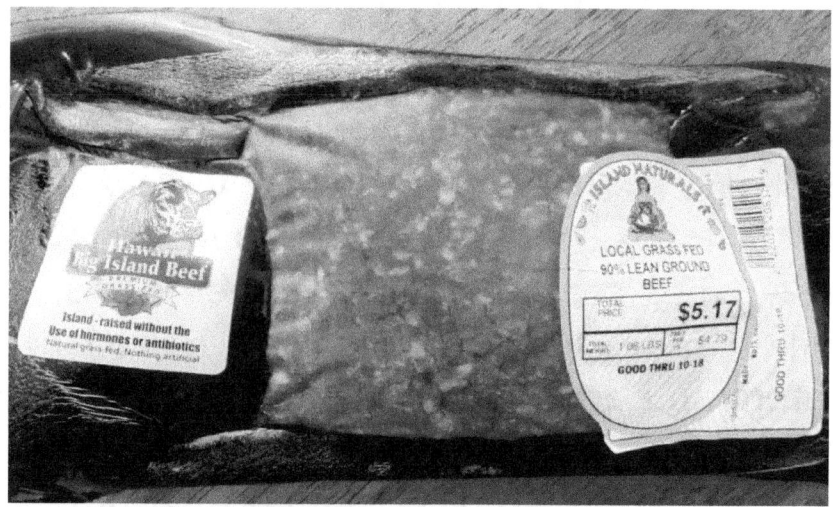

Hawaii Island raised grass-fed beef

Grass-fed beef is different than grain-fed beef. It has less fat, more omega-3 fatty acids, more conjugated linoleic acid (CLA), and more antioxidant vitamins such as Vitamin E.[7]

Hawaii Island beef has become a major part of our low-carbohydrate diet. When we first started eating grass-fed beef, we noticed it was tougher and tasted different than the grain-fed beef. We have become accustomed to the taste and now prefer it. Part of the challenge was learning how to cook it. The lower fat content of grass-fed beef makes it tough if it is overcooked. We add fat or coconut oil to keep it from drying out when cooking it in a pan. We slice it thin to avoid overcooking it on a grill. We also let the beef rest 10 to 15 minutes before serving it which lets the juices settle.

Hawaii Island ground beef is available for $5 or less a pound and steak for $8 to $12 a pound making it an affordable and healthy meal.

Are locally grown vegetables better?

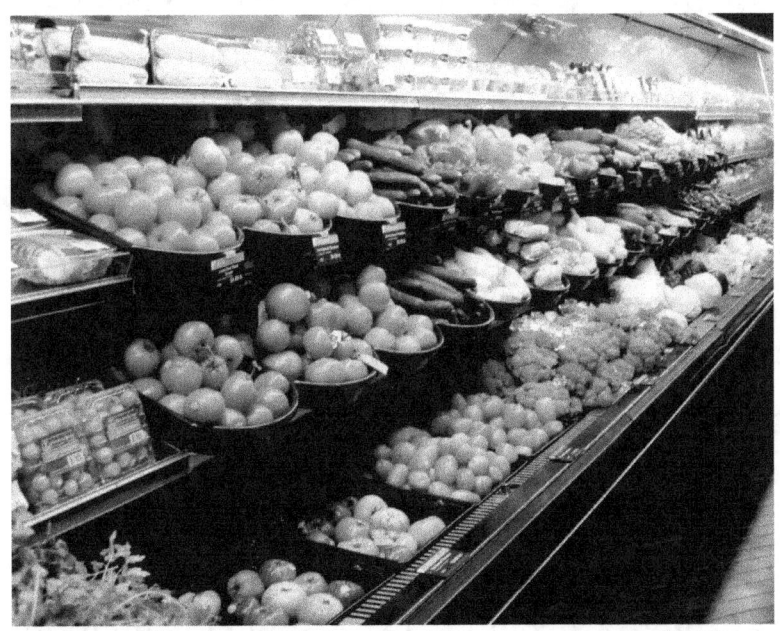

Hawaii vegetables in the grocery store

Farmer's markets in Hawaii have a large selection of locally grown vegetables, nuts, fruits, flowers, and food products. The variety and year round availability of produce makes it possible to live entirely on fresh, locally grown foods.

Vegetables harvested at their peak of maturity tend to have the most nutrients. Unless fruits or vegetables are frozen, dried, or canned they slowly lose their moisture, oxidize, and spoil after being harvested.[8] Many of the farms in Hawaii are organic which results in higher levels of antioxidants with less pesticide residue in fruits and vegetables as compared to conventionally grown produce. When we go to local Farmer's markets we ask the vendors if they actually grew the produce and how recently they were picked. We eat fresh vegetables as soon as possible after we buy them.

The amazing variety of delicious vegetables grown in Hawaii include avocados, ginger, bitter melon, cabbage, cucumber, radish (daikon), eggplant, lettuce, spinach, fiddlehead fern (warabi), tomatoes, broccoli, cauliflower, sweet potatoes, and mushrooms. You can also find asparagus, artichoke, beans, beets, burdock, carrots, celery, onion, peppers, pumpkin, radish, watercress, zucchini, basil, chives, cilantro, dill, lemongrass, mint, oregano, parsley, rosemary, and sage.[9]

Farmer's Markets and local grocery stores are an adventure with so many choices in lettuces, tomatoes, and colorful vegetables. There are over 110 types of avocados just on Hawaii Island in different shapes and sizes. Every type has a very different taste. We make a salad most evenings from locally grown lettuces, tomatoes, cucumbers, avocados, and any other vegetables that look good.

Macadamia nuts are a highly nutritious tropical nut grown in Hawaii. The nut is packed with nutrients including vitamin A, vitamin E, B-6 thiamin, riboflavin, niacin, and folates as well as moderate amounts of zinc, copper, iron, calcium, phosphorus, potassium, manganese, selenium, and magnesium. Macadamia nuts are unique with healthy oleic and palmitoleic fatty acids. We eat the nuts as high-fiber snacks and grind them into flour to make non-wheat "biscuits" and pie crusts.

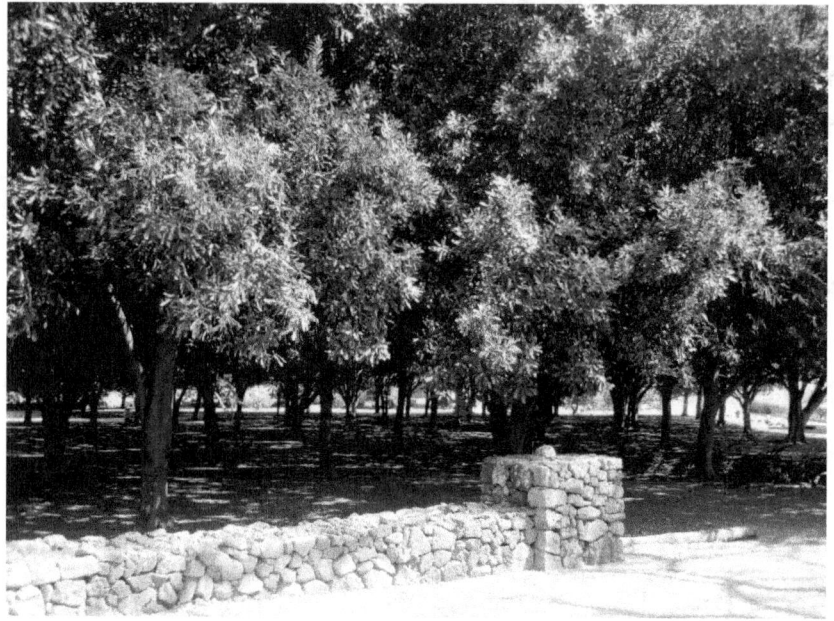

Macadamia nut grove in Hawaii

Although Hawaii has an abundance of sweet, tropical fruits, we eat very little fruit in order to keep our sugar and carbohydrates low.

Having a huge variety of locally grown vegetables available all year has dramatically changed what we eat and how we shop. Instead of stocking up on frozen meals, we shop several times a week to get the freshest produce, fish, and meats.

Can local Hawaii foods help you lose weight?

When we talk to visitors in Hawaii, they often tell us they feel so much better. Although the sun and warmth are a big factor, they tell us they are eating differently than they normally do at home on the mainland. In addition to eating more fish, grass-fed beef, and fresh vegetables one of the big differences in the Hawaii diet is the substitution of rice for bread.

People in Hawaii eat an average of 100 pounds of rice a year as compared to Americans on the mainland who eat only 26 pounds a year.[10] Rice is offered with eggs for breakfast and next to kimchee, warabi, or limu salad (seaweed) on local plate-lunches. *Loco Moco*, which is rice topped with a hamburger patty, egg, and gravy, was invented in Hilo and is available at drive-ins and fast-food joints throughout the state. Hilo's Café 100 sells over 9000 Loco Moco's a month. *Musubi*, which is rice wrapped in seaweed, is a snack or entire meal on the run and as convenient as a sandwich.

Bread is extremely expensive in Hawaii because it has to be shipped long distances. It is old and often stale by the time it reaches Hawaii's local grocery store shelves. Local bakeries have to include the high cost of electricity in their price. Rice is much cheaper than other grains and it is easier to store in Hawaii's heat and humidity. Though rice is a carbohydrate with a high glycemic index, it is less processed than wheat flour with no extra chemicals like bromine added. Many people find they eat fewer calories and feel fuller longer when eating rice instead of bread.

We ate less bread after moving to Hawaii because of the high cost, however, we stopped eating it entirely after reading studies about the negative health effects of wheat. According to Dr. Perlmutter, eating wheat products, even organic whole-grain wheat, makes you hungry, fat, and destroys your brain.[11] The starch in bread is absorbed so rapidly into the blood stream that it causes a huge spike in insulin which has side effects like arthritis, diabetes, and heart disease. Even when eating a low calorie diet, the calories from bread are stored as fat.

This explained why we struggled to lose weight on very low calorie diets that included low-fat breads and tortillas. We had already taken sugar out of our diet to reduce inflammation in order to control gout. It had not occurred to us that bread acts like sugar and can also cause gout attacks. Since removing wheat from our diet Tyler has not had any gout attacks.

Another benefit of going wheat free has been the savings on our grocery bill. Processed foods like breakfast cereals, pizzas, and frozen meals shipped from the mainland are very expensive in Hawaii. It is cheaper to buy a pound of local beef or fish than a box of cereal.

Having excellent health is more than just what you eat, it is also what you don't eat. In Hawaii, it is easy to make major changes in your diet because of the nutritious foods that are readily available year round and the non-standard diet on the island.

References

1. D. Mozaffarian, "Fish and n-3 fatty acids for the prevention of fatal coronary heart disease and sudden cardiac death," *American Journal of Clinical Nutrition* 87, no. 6 (2008):1991S-1996S.
2. K. He and others, "Accumulated evidence on fish consumption and coronary heart disease mortality: a meta-analysis of cohort studies," *Circulation* 109, no. 22 (2004): 2705-2711.
3. E. J. Schaefer and others, "Plasma phosphatidylcholine docosahexaenoic acid content and risk of dementia and Alzheimer disease: the Framingham Heart Study," *Archives of Neurology* 63, no. 11 (2006): 1545-1550.
4. J. K. Virtanen and others, "Fish consumption and risk of subclinical brain abnormalities on MRI in older adults," *Neurology*, 71, no. 6 (2008): 439-446.
5. Cristina Augood and others, "Oily fish consumption, dietary docosahexaenoic acid and eicosapentaenoic acid intakes, and associations with neovascular age-related macular

degeneration," *American Journal of Clinical Nutrition* 88, no. 2 (2008):398-406.

6. D. Mozaffarian and E. B. Rimm, "Fish intake, contaminants, and human health: evaluating the risks and the benefits," *JAMA* 296, no. 15 (2006): 1885-99.

7. Jo Johnson, "Why Grassfed is Best!," website: http://www.americangrassfedbeef.com/grass-fed-natural-beef.asp
last accessed 12/1/2014.

8. Joy Rickman, Diane Barrett, and Christine Bruhn, "Nutritional comparison of fresh, frozen, and canned fruits and vegetables," *Journal of the Science of Food and Agriculture* 87,no.6 (2007):930-944.

9. Hilo Farmer's Market, website: http://hilofarmersmarket.com
last accessed 12/1/2014.

10. CULCON, "Major US Crops: Rice," *Cross Currents*, (2003), website: http://www.crosscurrents.hawaii.edu/content.aspx?lang=eng&site=us&theme=work&subtheme=AGRIC&unit=USWORK043
last accessed 12/1/2014.

11. David Perlmutter, *Grain Brain: The Surprising Truth about Wheat, Carbs, and Sugar--Your Brain's Silent Killers* (New York: Little Brown and Company, 2013).

Chapter Six
ACTIVE OUTDOOR LIFESTYLE

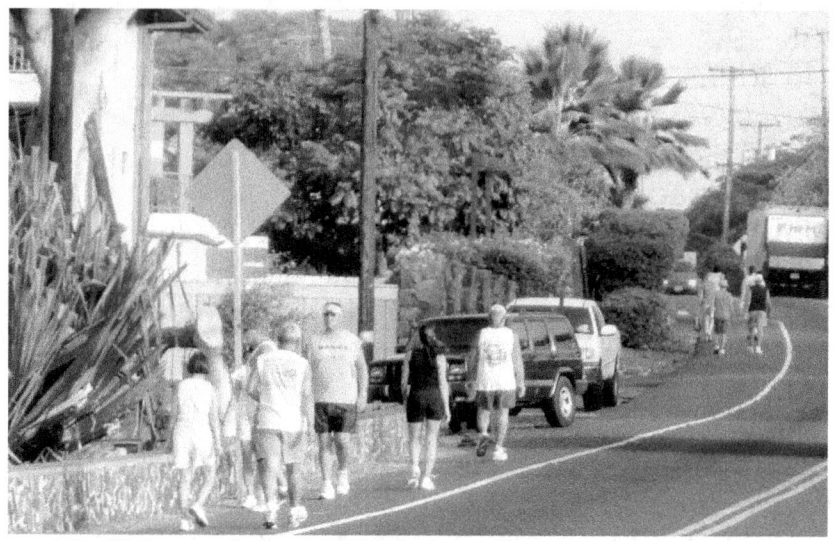

Walking along Alii Drive in Kona, Hawaii

Hawaii's warm, sunny weather makes it easy to be active and out in nature every day of the year. It is not unusual to see people on the beach in their 80's and 90's with remarkable health and fitness. Hawaii's climate and gorgeous scenery inspires an active outdoor lifestyle.

On our vacations to Hawaii we were energized after a few days outside in the sun. We were able to wake up early for a morning walk, swim during the day, and take another walk in the evening. This was far more activity than usual for us and we felt so good that we would promise ourselves that we would keep up the extra exercise when we returned home to the mainland. Our resolve never lasted more than a month in the cold, dark winter weather. A walk in the cold rain made us feel tired and miserable instead of energized.

Can you exercise your fat off?

After we moved to Hawaii, our plan was to quickly lose weight by eating healthy foods and burning calories with lots of exercise. We assumed we could spend all of our free time exercising and our fat would just melt away.

We did the "calorie math" to figure out how much exercise we needed to do each day to lose two pounds a week. We calculated that we needed to exercise 500 calories a day just to lose a pound a week (based on the theory that a pound of fat is equal to 3500 calories). We joined a water aerobics class and also walked every day, two exercises that we were able to manage in our obese state. We were surprised at the paltry number of calories we were able to burn off considering the effort and exhaustion. After 45 minutes of water aerobics (250 calories) and 45 minutes of walking (200 calories) we were sore, hungry, and needed a long nap.

During our first year in Hawaii, we learned that at our age it was impossible for us to exercise off our fat. Our only option for losing weight was by changing our diet. As we reduced our calories, we were shocked at how few calories we needed to eat to lose weight. The on-line calculators that publish basal metabolic rates (BMR), the amount of calories a person burns without doing anything, were completely wrong for us. We could gain weight eating our BMR amount of calories even with exercise.

Although the rising obesity rate in the United States is constantly blamed on low activity levels, research contradicts the claim that lack of exercise is responsible. A study of the Hadza tribe of hunter-gatherers in Tanzania compared their activity and metabolism with Westerners.[1] Although the Hadza had more physical activity, the average amount of calories they burned during the day was no different than an average Westerner. The finding that metabolic rates are similar between very fit hunter-gather tribe members and less active Westerners helps to explain why exercise is not the solution to obesity. Diet is the only way to combat being overweight.

Other studies that have tried to explain why exercise does not result in weight loss have concluded that exercise burns only a small amount of energy while at the same time greatly increasing hunger and the calories eaten, particularly for women.[2,3] One surprising study showed that metabolism is not actually increased by more activity as we have been told. In fact, basal metabolic rates (BMRs) actually drop as a person loses weight.[4] The Pennington Biomedical Research Center created a weight loss predictor that takes into consideration a person's "metabolic adaption" based on their age, height, gender, and current weight.[5]

Our experience with dieting confirms the study's finding that the body burns less calories as you lose weight. We had to continually cut our calories to keep losing. On a low-calorie diet, our hunger pangs would always get the best of us and we would always gain some our weight back. Our exercise routine made us hungry and unable to keep from eating more.   It seemed like an impossible struggle.

It was only when we gave up counting calories and switched to a low-carbohydrate diet that we were able to lose weight and keep it off.   The low-carbohydrate, or ketogenic diet, stopped our constant hunger and seesawing weight change.   We also discovered that moderate exercise did not make us sore or increase our appetite and less exercise left us with energy to accomplish other things during the day.

Moderate exercise has been shown to actually curb your appetite, as compared to high-intensity exercise that causes you to eat more and be more inactive the rest of the day. [6,7] We were less hungry after an uplifting walk for 20 minutes as compared to 45 minutes of water aerobics.

When we stopped trying to exercise off our fat, we focused on outdoor activities that we found enjoyable. We walk every day on a coastal path that we find uplifting and beautiful. We stop and enjoy the view and sit next to the crashing waves. We swim and snorkel with friends. Now we exercise because it makes us feel great rather than to burn calories.

Does moderate exercise make you healthier?

Though exercise may not lead to weight loss, there are many other health benefits. Exercise helps the immune system fight off bacterial and viral infections and it helps prevent diabetes, hypertension, cardiovascular heart disease, osteoporosis, depression, and some forms of cancer. [8] A study by Dr. Andersen and Swedish researchers found that just one hour of moderate exercise a day is enough to reduce the risk of heart failure by 46%.[9]

A large clinical trial at the University of Pittsburgh showed that moderate physical activity can help older people stay mobile and independent.[10] The two year exercise program consisted of walking for 150 minutes a week and strength exercises from a seated position. The activity helped aging adults maintain their ability to walk as compared to other older adults who did not exercise.

You get the benefits of exercise whether you do it all at one time or in several short sessions.[11] Fortunately, the temperatures in Hawaii barely fluctuate all year so we spread our activity between the early morning and late afternoon to avoid the heat of the day.

Is sweating good for you?

Another benefit of being physically active is sweating. When we lived on the mainland we went to saunas during the winter. We had heard about the mercury miners in Spain reducing the effects of their exposure to mercury vapor by taking saunas. Although we were only able to go occasionally, we always felt better after removing toxins by sweating.

In Hawaii it is easy to sweat during the day and get the detoxifying effect. Many toxic elements are eliminated more readily through sweat. Toxic chemicals such as phthalates in plastics, bisphenol A (BPA), arsenic, cadmium, lead, and mercury are found in sweat.[13] Researchers theorize that some toxins are stored in tissues and therefore more easily eliminated through sweat.[12]

Chinese researchers determined that sweat is a good way to eliminate urea from the body. Urea is created when the body metabolizes protein and is primarily eliminated by the kidneys. Though urea is not considered extremely toxic, sweating helps take the pressure off the kidneys that flush it out of the body. The researchers also found that sweat eliminates only a little uric acid. It is important to drink a lot of fluids when sweating to keep the levels of uric acid from increasing in the blood.[14] Tyler learned this the hard way after getting a gout attack from being overheated and dehydrated.

Does being outdoors make you feel happier?

Spending time in nature has been shown to make people more relaxed, calm, and happy. A Japanese research team at Chiba University found that sounds of nature, like the sound of water flowing in a river, changed the brain blood flow to a state of relaxation. Another study at Stockholm University found that nature sounds calmed people whereas road traffic noise measurably increased their stress. Research published in *Psychological*

Medicine showed that hearing bird songs lifts the mood and decreases fatigue. Research at Wheeling Jesuit University found that the aromatic chemicals in flowers can increase alertness, even in extremely small amounts.[15]

Hawaii's ocean, colorful flowers, trees, and birds make it easy to have an active outdoor lifestyle. The sounds of wind blowing through the palm leaves, the sweet scent of tropical flowers, and the sound of the crashing waves on our walks put us into a calm and joyful state.

Do you live longer with an active lifestyle?

Being fit or active has been shown to reduce the risk of death from any cause by more than 50%. Increasing your level of physical activity by just 1000 calories a week (equal to about 5 hours of walking) has been shown to lower risk of death by 20% to 35%. In contrast, physically inactive middle-aged women were shown to have a 52% increase in all causes of death compared to physically active women.[8]

We always struggled to walk regularly during the cold, overcast winters on the mainland but in Hawaii getting a moderate amount of exercise to help prolong our life feels effortless.

It does not take extreme activity to gain the benefits of exercise, just consistency. A study of exercise habits among a group of 416,175 Taiwanese adults showed that only 15 minutes of moderate exercise a day (92 minutes a week) increased their life span by about three years and decreased their risk of death from any cause by about 14%. In the study, the participants who started more ambitious exercise programs gained some additional risk reduction, but the benefits reached a plateau quickly. Each additional 15 minutes a day of moderate exercise decreased their risk of death by only another 4%.[16]

Living in Hawaii, with perfect weather and gorgeous scenery makes it easy to keep active all year round. The increased activity of people in Hawaii helps explain why the islands' residents are healthier and live longer lives.

References

1. H. Pontze and others, "Hunter-Gatherer Energetics and Human Obesity," *PLoS ONE* 1371 (2012): e40503.

2. T. A. Hagobian and others, "Effects of exercise on energy-regulating hormones and appetite in men and women," *American Journal of Physiology* 296, no. 2 (2009):R233-42.

3. M. Pomerleau and others, "Effects of exercise intensity on food intake and appetite in women," *American Journal of Clinical Nutrition* 80, no 5 (2004): 1230-6.

4. D. M Thomas and others, "Why do individuals not lose more weight from an exercise intervention at a defined dose? An energy balance analysis," *Obesity Review* 13, no. 10 (2012): 835-47.

5. Pennington Biomedical Research Center, "weight loss predictor," website: http://www.pbrc.edu/research-and-faculty/calculators/weight-loss-predictor last accessed 12/1/2014.

6. C. Martins and others, "Effects of exercise on gut peptides, energy intake and appetite," *Journal of Endocrinology* 193, no. 2 (2007):251-8.

7. M. Rosenkilde and others, "Body fat loss and compensatory mechanisms in response to different doses of aerobic exercise--a randomized controlled trial in overweight sedentary males," *American Journal of Physiology Regulatory, Integrative and Comparative Physiology* 303, no. 6 (2012):R571-9.

8. D. E. Warburton, C. W. Nicol, and S. S. Bredin, "Health benefits of physical activity: the evidence," *Canadian Medical Association Journal* 174, no. 6 (2006): 801-809.

9. K. Andersen and others, "Dose-response relationship of total and leisure time physical activity to risk of heart failure: a prospective cohort study," *Circulation: Heart Failure* 7, no. 5 (2014): 701-8.

10. Jack Kelly, "Moderate exercising beneficial to the aging, Study proves daily exercise can prevent loss of mobility," *Pittsburgh Post-Gazette* May 27, 2014.

11. J. Jakicic and others, "Prescribing exercise in multiple short bouts versus one continuous bout: effects on adherence, cardiorespiratory fitness, and weight loss in overweight women," *International Journal of Obesity Related Metabolic Disorders* 19, no. 12 (1995): 893-901.

12. Stephen Genuis and others, "Blood, Urine, and Sweat (BUS) Study: Monitoring and Elimination of Bioaccumulated Toxic Elements," *Archives of Environmental Contamination and Toxicology* 61, no. 2 (2011): 344-357.

13. M. Sears, K. Kerr, and R. Bray, "Arsenic, Cadmium, Lead, and Mercury in Sweat: A Systematic Review," *Journal of Environmental and Public Health* 2012 (2012): 184745.

14. C. T. Huang and others, "Uric acid and urea in human sweat," *Chinese Journal of Physiology* 45, no. 3 (2002): 109-15.

15 Eva Selhub and Alan Logan, *Your Brain on Nature: The Science of Nature's Influence on Your Health, Happiness, and Vitality* (Canada: Wiley 2012).

16. C. P. Wen and others, "Minimum amount of physical activity for reduced mortality and extended life expectancy: a prospective cohort study," *The Lancet* 378, no. 9798 (2011): 1244-1253.

Chapter Seven
SLOW PACE OF LIFE

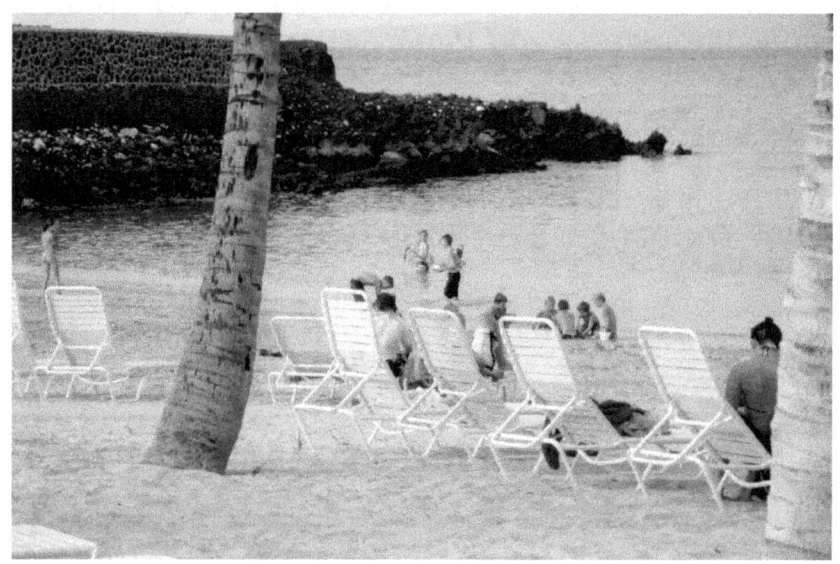

Relaxing in Hawaii

The pace of everything is slower in Hawaii and after slowing down for a while it starts to feel very good. We moved to Hawaii to escape our stressful life. As we relaxed and began to enjoy the warm weather, ocean breezes, fragrant flowers, and delicious food, our personalities changed. We became more easy-going, talked slower, slept more, and worried less.

Stress causes the adrenal glands to produce the cortisol hormone. Cortisol makes energy available by blocking insulin, keeping glucose circulating in the blood, and suppressing the immune system. High levels of cortisol for long periods of time causes serious health problems including digestive problems, heart disease, anxiety, depression, weight gain, and concentration problems.

Lack of sleep, lack of exercise, too much caffeine, and lack of nutrition can all contribute to stress and increase cortisol levels. Long term stress can make you fat, sick, and ultimately shorten your life.

Does slowing down improve your health?

In Hawaii, people take the time to read, relax, and smell the flowers. People drive, eat, and walk slower than people living in big cities on the mainland. The "time is money" reality doesn't exist; the stock market action and news cycles are over before lunch. Living a relaxed thoughtful life, with time to sit on the beach, listen to the birds, and take a nap melts away our stress and worry.

A Dutch study showed that people with easy-going personalities have more healthy lifestyles including more physical activity and a balanced diet. They also consume less alcohol, coffee, and tobacco.[1] As we have slowed the pace of our life, we have also adopted more healthy habits. We have more time to concentrate on our nutrition and what we eat. We have been able to stop drinking coffee which was really a surprise to us.

Not everyone enjoys the slower pace of life in Hawaii. We have met many people who became so frustrated with slow service, lack of high paying jobs, or their inability to change things after moving to Hawaii that they moved back to the mainland. For some, the desire for prestige and accomplishment are more important than a slow pace of life.

In a study published in the *Journal of Applied Psychology* about the consequences of ambition, researchers found that while "go-getters" are more likely to attend prestigious universities and have high-paying jobs, they are only slightly happier than their less-ambitious counterparts and they live shorter lives.[2] For the study, Notre Dame researchers followed over 700 "high-ability" people over several decades, from college until retirement age. The participants were surveyed at certain points in their lives to measure how satisfied they were in their occupation, family life, leisure activities, health, and 'joy in living'. The majority were surveyed in their mid-50's at the peak of their careers.

The study on the consequences of ambition indicated that ambition was strongly correlated with high educational attainment, occupation prestige, and income. Unfortunately, these same accomplishments were not helpful in increasing happiness and longevity. Those who were identified as the most ambitious had a 15.5% higher mortality rate by the end of the study than those who were the least ambitious. The effect was worse among ambitious people who did not achieve the success they were striving for.

There have been times in our life when our ambitions and achievements were more important to us than our health. In our experience you can slow down the pace of your life even after years of being a "go getter" and embrace a slower paced and healthier way of living.

Does socialization help you live longer?

One of the benefits of a slower pace of life is that there is more time to socialize. People gather frequently in Hawaii to share food and "talk story". Stories are told of a recent hike or beautiful fish encountered while snorkeling. When checking out at the grocery store, we often wait patiently as the clerk talks story with a customer. Talking is a way of life on the islands and stories are so quickly spread it is called the "coconut wireless". The quality and number of a person's social relationships have been linked to their mental health, illness, and longevity.

A study at the Centre for Ageing Studies at Flinders University followed nearly 1,500 older people for 10 years and found that those with a large network of friends outlived those with the fewest friends by 22%.[3] The researchers concluded that friends discourage unhealthy behaviors such as smoking and heavy drinking and may prevent depression, improve self-esteem, and provide support. Interestingly, having close relationships with children and relatives had no effect on longevity.

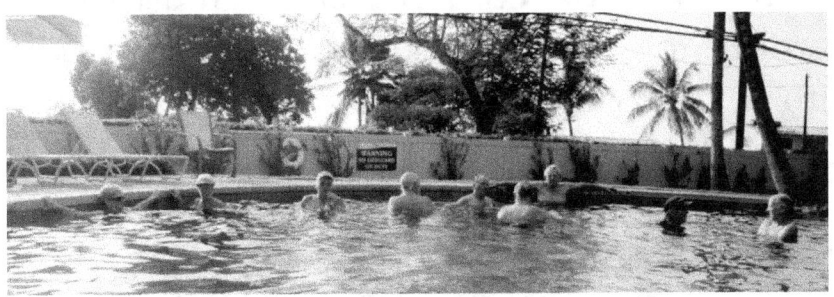

Socializing in Kona, Hawaii

Another study by Fabsitz showed that people who do not participate in group activities and have no social support have a higher risk of sleep problems.[5] Lack of sleep has been shown to cause serious health problems over time.[6] It can also cause depression, weight gain, memory problems, and accidents. British researchers investigated how sleep patterns affected the mortality of 10,000 civil servants over two decades. Their results showed that a lack of sleep increases the risk of death, however, too much sleep also increases the risk of death. Higher rates of all causes of death existed among participants who reported short sleep times (5 hours or less) or long sleep times (9 hours or more). Getting less sleep was associated with a 110% excess risk of cardiovascular mortality. Getting too much sleep was associated with a 110% excess risk of death by other causes.[6]

In Okinawa Japan, women who live the longest belong to "moai" groups, friends who meet about once a week to walk, have a potluck, or do some other activity. When 300 moai groups of 6 to 8 people each were formed in Minnesota, the collective groups lost 76,000 pounds and added 3.2 years of life expectancy after four years of meetings.[4]

Are islands associated with longevity?

The small Greek island of Ikaria has been identified as one of the "blue zones" by author Dan Buettner where the residents live an average of 10 years longer than the rest of Western Europe.[4] Other clusters of people who have great longevity, or blue zones, include the island of Okinawa in Japan and a group of mountain villages on the island of Sardinia in Italy. Many of the attributes of island living on Ikaria including the friendly, active lifestyle and eating locally grown foods are similar to living on the islands in Hawaii.

Buettner and blue zone researchers believe other elements of lifestyle are also significant to longevity including having a tight knit community with similar values that is willing to accept you and a laid back culture where no one is in a hurry.[4]

It is easier to grow old in blue zone cultures that do not emphasize youth and value the elderly and their contributions.[4] A sense of purpose, feeling valued and supported by the community, being active and doing meaningful activities helps you to live long and enjoy life. Elderly people, called *kupuna*, are respected in Hawaii and sought after by the community for volunteer work, teaching, and other jobs.

The pace of life in blue zones is slow, people socialize frequently, and mid-day naps are the norm. Other reasons given for the clusters of longevity are behaviors such as limiting calorie intake, not smoking, drinking moderate amounts of wine, and staying active.[4]

For us, making lifestyle changes to improve our health have been difficult, even with intensive effort. Living in Hawaii we were able to make seemingly impossible changes to our lifestyle, slow the pace of our life, and get healthy.

References

1. L. Koppes, J. Snel and H. Kemper, "Personality, a determinant of lifestyle?," *Amsterdam Growth and Health Longitude Study: A 23 Year Follow-up from Teenager to Adult about Lifestyle and Health* 47 (2004): 132-143.

2. T. Judge and J. Kammeyer-Mueler, "On the value of aiming high: the causes and consequences of ambition," *Journal of Applied Psychology* 97, no. 4 (2012):758-75.

3. J. Holt-Lunstad, T. Smith, and J. Layton, "Social Relationships and Mortality Risk: A Meta-analytic Review," *PLOS Medicine* 7, no. 7 (2010): e1000316.

4. Dan Buettner, *The Blue Zones: Lessons for Living Longer from the People Who've Lived the Longest,* (Washington D.C.: National Geographic, 2010).

5. R. Fabsitz, P. Sholinsky, and J. Goldberg, "Correlates of sleep problems among men: the Vietnam Era Twin Registry," *Journal of Sleep Research* 6, no. 1 (1997): 50-56.

6. Jane Ferrie and others, "A prospective study of change in sleep duration; associations with mortality in the Whitehall II Cohort," *Sleep* 30, no. 12 (2007):1659-1666.

Chapter Eight
HEALTHY HOME

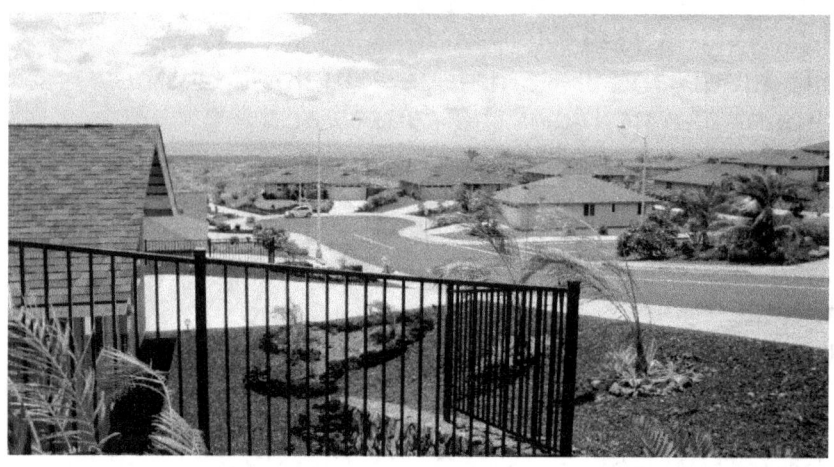

The community, neighborhood, and home you live in can greatly contribute to your health and wellbeing. Getting a good deal on a rental or home purchase in an area with dreary weather or a run-down neighborhood may affect your safety, health, and longevity.

Can your neighborhood impact health?

Studies have shown that the characteristics of your neighborhood are related to your health and well-being. A European study by Dr. Ellaway showed that in neighborhoods with a lot of greenery residents were over three times more likely to be to be physically active than other neighborhoods.[1]

Studies of residents in deteriorated neighborhoods with abandoned cars, litter, graffiti, and homes in disrepair have higher rates of disease, murder, and early death, regardless of their income.[2] Residents in neighborhoods with a large number of boarded-up vacant housing units have higher rates of premature death from all causes including diabetes, homicide, and suicide.[3] Residents in neighborhoods where the houses and gardens are maintained, garbage is picked up, graffiti is painted over, and kids are watched have lower rates of disease, murder, and suicide compared to deteriorated neighborhoods, regardless of the residents' income or race.[3]

Hawaii has many types of neighborhoods from very upscale to poor areas. The healthiest places to live are in the communities that care about their homes, public spaces, and where residents are respectful to their neighbors. In Hawaii people talk about caring for the land, *malama ʻaina*, but the evidence of their care varies greatly.

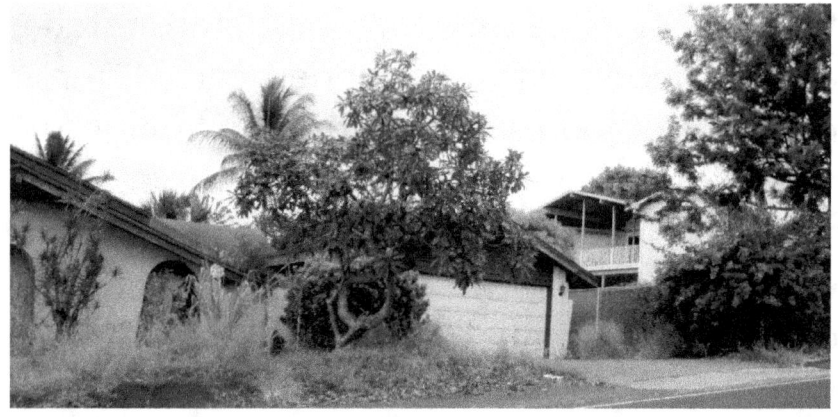

Can your neighborhood make you fat?

Studies have shown that in deteriorated neighborhoods with litter, graffiti, filth and a lack of greenery, residents are 50% more likely to be overweight or obese.[1] However, living within a half-mile of healthy food outlets is related to lower rates of obesity.[5] Studies by Rand Corp found that people who lived within one mile of parks, playgrounds, walking paths, and running tracks were more physically active.[6] Having four or more different types of businesses in the neighborhood and four-way intersections increases the number of walking trips among residents.[7] The age of the neighborhood, availability of parking, and block lengths have not been shown to affect the amount of walking.

When searching for a new home, we look for sidewalks, crosswalks, parks, Farmer's markets and grocery stores within walking distance to the neighborhood. The environment and people living around you affect you every day and affect your weight.

Some interesting research by Dr. Christakis shows how obesity can spread through a network of friends.[8] After evaluating a large social network of more than 12,000 people over 32 years the study showed that a person's chances of becoming obese increased by 57% if they had a friend who became obese. If a sibling became obese the person's chance of becoming obese increased by 40% and if their spouse became obese it increased by 37%.

When you live around people dedicated to keeping their neighborhood safe and you have friends who are active and fit, it increases your likelihood of being healthy, active, and fit. When we lived in Kona, we were surrounded by super fit athletes in the neighborhood constantly preparing for Ironman competitions. The presence of the athletes around the neighborhood seemed to encourage elderly couples to walk, run, and swim in the ocean and they in turn inspired us to be more active.

Does your neighborhood have a history?

When looking at a neighborhood, we check maps and historical records to make sure the area was not previously used as a chemical waste dump or downwind from a plant releasing contaminates. Hawaii has some superfund sites that the EPA is tracking for cleanup such as the Geothermal Vent in Puna, the Pioneer Mill Company in Lahaina, the Naval complex in

Pearl Harbor, the Village of Kunia on Oahu, and Schofield Barracks in Wahiawa. The Hawaii State Department of Health publishes a list of sites with potential or known hazardous substances, pollutants, or contaminants called the *128D Hawaii State Response Program Site List* every year along with the DOD Program List of Priority Sites.[9]

Unfortunately, Hawaii's agricultural industry uses a lot of pesticides and herbicides on their crops. Nearby farms and pastures can contaminate the air and water. A report by the Hawaii State Department of Agriculture stated that Hawaii uses pesticides at a rate 10 times higher than the national average.[10] An example of one of the contaminated sites is Walker Bay on Oahu which was once used by a sugar company to mix pesticide and herbicide solutions to spray on sugar cane fields. Measurements of dioxins and furans at the site, which are highly toxic and persistent chemicals, were well above safe soil levels for residential areas based on EPA standards.

Hawaii also has contamination from military training activities that have left toxic waste and "depleted" uranium from target practice. Military bases and training sites have petroleum, oils, lubricants, lead, asbestos, PCBs, and hazardous wastes left in the soil. Fortunately, Hawaii has never had much heavy industry and since land is limited developers often agree to clean it up as a part of their development costs.

Although we research areas the best we can before moving, we have had to make peace with living in the toxic world. We take adequate precautions based on contaminants we know about in the neighborhood and then stop worrying about it.

We moved to a neighborhood in California located next to a superfund site that had been remediated for toxic compounds in the ground water due to improper handling of hazardous waste. Knowing that the ground water was an issue, we installed a water filter and RO filter before moving into the house.

Can your home help you live longer?

A home in Hawaii can improve your health and extend your life or do the opposite. Large windows that open to let fresh air flow through the house and keep you from overheating can keep you healthy. Living in a house with mold, mildew, dry rot, termites, or bug infestations can be stressful and unhealthy.

When we lived in Hilo we were enchanted with the lush grass and fruit trees. We tried to keep our environment as free of toxins as possible, but the reality is that it is difficult to live in the tropics without herbicides and pesticides to deal with the onslaught of bugs. Taking care of the endlessly growing grass and year round fruit production was exhausting. We were happier living in a condo where we could enjoy the tropical gardens being maintained by gardeners paid by home owners fees.

When selecting a home, we make sure it is not in a flood zone or near standing water that can breed mosquitoes. Many people have been upset to find their homes are downwind of the volcano with frequent choking vog (volcanic emissions), in a dangerous lava zone area, or at risk for being destroyed by a tsunami.

You can find more details about what to look for in a Hawaii house in our book, *Your Ideal Hawaii Home*: *Avoid Disaster when Buying or Building in Hawaii.*

References

1. A. Ellaway, S. Macintyre, and X. Bonnefoy, "Graffiti, greenery, and obesity in adults: secondary analysis of European cross sectional survey,". *BMJ*. 331 no. 7517 (2005): 611–2.
2. D. Cohen and others, "Neighborhood Physical Conditions and Health," *American Journal of Public Health* 93, no. 3 (2003): 467-471.
3. D. Cohen and others, "Contribution of Public Parks to Physical Activity," *American Journal of Public Health* 97, no. 3 (2007): 509–514.
4. T. Glass, M. Rasmussen, and B. Schwartz, "Neighborhoods and Obesity in Older Adults: The Baltimore Memory Study," *American Journal of Preventative Medicine* 31, no. 6 (2006): 455-463.
5. A. Rundle and others, "Neighborhood Food Environment and Walkability Predict Obesity in New York City," *Environmental Health Perspectives* 117 (2009): 442-447.

6. D. Cohen and others, *Park Use and Physical Activity in a Sample of Public Parks in the City of Los Angeles* (Santa Monica: RAND Corporation, TR-357-HLTH, 2006).

7. Rob Boer and others, "Neighborhood Design and Walking Trips in Ten U.S. Metropolitan Areas," *American Journal of Preventive Medicine* 32, no. 4 (2007): 298–304.

8. N. A. Christakis and J. H. Fowler, "The Spread of Obesity in a Large Social Network Over 32 Years," *New England Journal of Medicine* 357, No. 4 (2007): 370-379.

9. Hawaii Department of Health, *Report to the Twenty-seventh Legislature State of Hawaii – Pursuant to Chapters 128D and 128E, Hawaii Revised Statutes Requiring the Department of Health to Report Environmental Response Laws and Hawaii Emergency Planning and Community Right to Know Act Financial and Environmental Site Information FY2013*, 2014.

10. State of Hawaii, Department of Agriculture. *Evaluation of Pesticide Problems in Hawaii* (Honolulu: Department of Agriculture State of Hawaii, 1969).

Chapter Nine
WHY THE BENEFITS MAY GO AWAY

We enjoy watching visitors and new residents become more active, vibrant, and healthy after spending time in Hawaii. It is disturbing to watch healthy people suddenly add 50 pounds of fat and complain of health issues that had previously disappeared. We came to realize the health benefits we get from living in Hawaii are from specific things we are doing, foods we are eating, and ways we are living in Hawaii's tropical climate. Even small changes in food or activities over time can reverse the benefits gained by living in Hawaii.

Can too much fruit be bad for you?

The amazing selection of delicious tropical fruits are inexpensive and available all year in Hawaii. Many people add a lot of fruit to their daily diet without thinking about the detrimental effects of eating that much sugar. Hawaii themed cocktails and sweets are also common at parties, potlucks, and restaurants making it easy to add a lot of sugar, specifically fructose, to your diet.

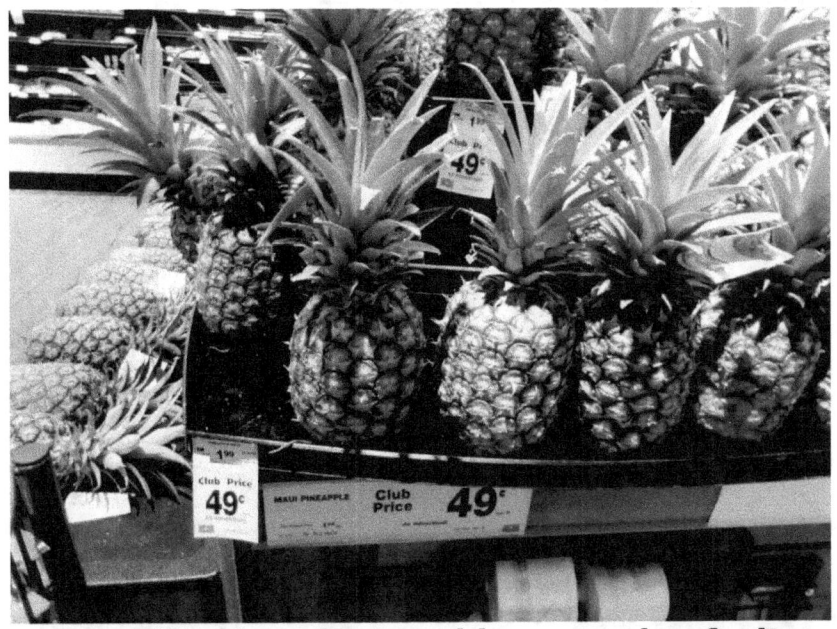

Hawaii's abundant and inexpensive fruit

Fructose, in fruit and corn syrup, has been found to cause a rise in uric acid levels which inflames the body. Eating a lot of fruit or sweeteners has been shown to cause "Metabolic Syndrome" which includes inflammation, increased blood pressure, insulin resistance, a rise in triglycerides, and an increase in fat.[1] Too much fructose can cause diabetes, gout, kidney disease, obesity, and non-alcoholic fatty liver disease.

What if old habits return?

Some people change their eating habits over time in Hawaii. When they first arrive they live on the fish, grass-fed beef, and local vegetables. They notice their weight loss and that they are feeling better. However, after a while they revert back to their previous way of living and eat mainland foods instead of local foods.

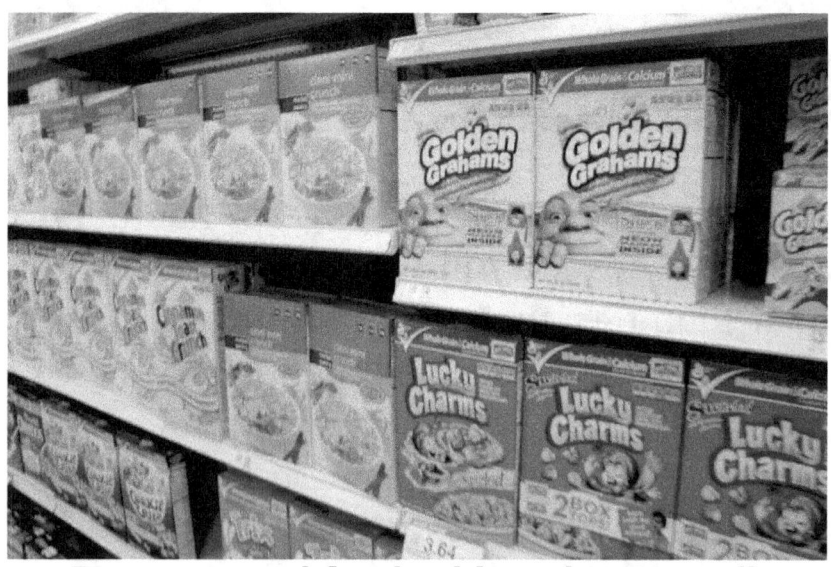

Preprocessed foods shipped to Hawaii

Over time, their weight increases and the health issues they left behind on the mainland return to them in Hawaii.

Can there be too many potlucks?

One of the top social pastimes in Hawaii is eating; a common island saying is "eat until you are tired". While living in Hilo and Kona we were invited to more parties and potlucks in a month than we were any year living on the mainland.

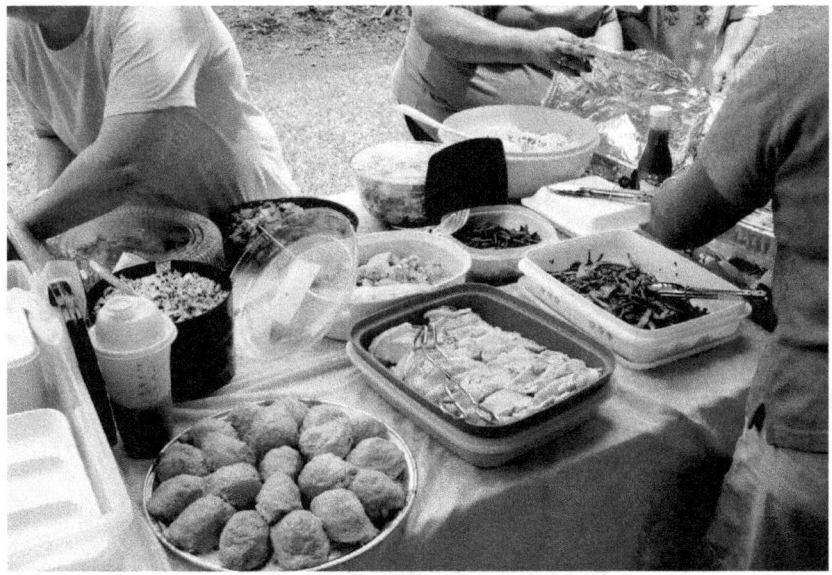

Hawaii style pot luck

Hawaii seems to attract gourmet cooks and at potlucks and parties it is common to have a huge banquet with the best tasting food imaginable. It takes incredible will power to keep from overeating. We find it very enjoyable to socialize but struggle to keep from overeating and regaining pounds we had worked for weeks to get off.

Can you be socially isolated in Hawaii?

Hawaii has the most social and accepting people we have ever met. However, people who cannot curb their condescending attitude, negativity, or intolerance can find themselves frustrated and isolated. Hawaii is very remote from the mainland and the time difference makes it harder to connect with family and friends far away. Boredom and loneliness can lead to depression, over drinking alcohol, and other unhealthy behaviors. Having friends with similar interests and goals helps us keep socially active and healthy.

Can you stay with complex medical needs?

Although Hawaii has excellent coverage for medical insurance, it is lacking in doctors and specialized care. Most serious medical problems on the outer islands require a trip to Oahu for hospital care or to see a specialized doctor. Some people regularly fly from the outer islands to Oahu for medical treatment.

We know of many elderly couples who left after living in Hawaii for over a decade because they wanted to be nearer to medical facilities or required long term care. Living in some places in Hawaii may not be feasible with certain health conditions because of a lack of facilities or doctors.

Do you need a sustainable passion?

We have learned that having a sustainable passion helps people stay engaged and optimistic. At a certain age surfing, motorcycle riding, tennis, or other athletic pursuits may no longer be possible. We have watched people decline when they no longer can pursue their physical passion. Less athletic activities like reading, writing, arts, crafts, or other pursuits can keep you sharp and happy. Living in Hawaii, we have had the benefit of plenty of time to learn and master new skills. Having a passion for writing, photography, and always learning has greatly added to the quality of our life

References

1. A. Miller and K. Adeli, "Dietary fructose and the metabolic syndrome," *Current Opinion in Gastroenterology* 24, no. 2 (2008): 204-9.

Chapter Ten
OUR HAWAII DIET

In our search for an answer to the mystery of why people are so healthy and happy in Hawaii, we started by researching the common activities and foods eaten in Hawaii. We did not realize how much nutrition there is in Hawaii's fish, local beef, vegetables, coconut oil, and seaweed nor how important the sunlight and ocean are to health. Just being in Hawaii improved our energy and feeling of well being. Making additional changes to our diet and adding supplements to increase our nutrition has improved our health even more. Our Hawaii diet is a low-carbohydrate diet with lots of saturated fats.

Although we have cited the medical studies that convinced us that our Hawaii diet is far healthier than the common American diet and verified the benefits of the diet ourselves, we are not doctors and have no medical training. The purpose of this book is to share the information and our personal experiences with others searching for ways to make healthy changes in their life.

The books and studies we cite by medical professionals to support the validity of our Hawaii diet are often in stark opposition to the recommendations of other medical authorities like the American Heart Association, publications by the government, and what has become the "common" health knowledge of our age. The Dietary Reference report published by the Institute of Medicine of the National Academies, for example, recommends that carbohydrates be 45 to 65% of the daily calories eaten.[1] That would be up to 243 grams of carbohydrates a day on a 1500 daily calorie diet (a gram of carbohydrate is 4 calories). We eat less than 50 grams a day of carbohydrates with the goal of always being in nutritional ketosis.

Nutritional ketosis is when the body burns ketones created from fat instead of glucose from carbohydrates. Living in ketosis, called the ketogenic diet, has been shown to reduce triglycerides, blood sugar, insulin levels, blood pressure, inflammation, and increase HDL levels. It also keeps us from being overwhelmed with hunger which allowed us to lose weight and maintain our weight loss without loss of energy or brain power.

To stay in ketosis, we eat no grains, sugar, or legumes. We avoid fruits and only eat small amounts of berries, lemons, and limes. We use urine test strips, called ketostix, on occasion to verify that we are in ketosis.

It can take up to a week to get into ketosis and adapt to burning ketones instead of glucose after starting a low carbohydrate diet. After adapting to a ketogenic diet, physical endurance returns as long as the diet has high amounts of fat (60% or more) and limits the amount of protein to 24% or less of the daily calories. [2]

We track every carbohydrate and eat only 30 to 50 grams a day or 120 to 200 calories maximum. The amount varies by person, Chris finds that she has to keep to 30 grams or less to stay in ketosis, whereas Tyler can eat up to 50 grams a day without a problem. We also track our overall calories to maintain our weight. We use our daily planner to keep track of what we eat and our weight each day. We publish *Your Ideal Hawaii Daily Planner* on Amazon each year.

Our Hawaii diet is composed of 60% saturated fats from coconut oil, beef, fish, pork, eggs, cheese, and butter. In contrast, the Institute of Medicine's report recommends linoleic acid (an omega-6 fatty acid) in unsaturated vegetable oils which we avoid completely.[1] Vegetable oils quickly turn rancid and form unhealthy trans fats even when lightly heated. We get plenty of omega-6 fatty acids in the eggs, cheese, and nuts. We get omega-3 fatty acids from fish and grass-fed beef. We are careful to not eat too much protein because excess amino acids created from protein will convert to glucose and take us out of ketosis. Our protein intake is calculated based on our desired weight at

1.2 grams of protein for every 2.2 pounds of body weight.

We get fiber in our diet from creamed coconut meat, nuts, berries, and low carbohydrate vegetables. We drink 1 quart of basic water for every 60 pounds of body weight and because we sweat a lot in Hawaii's hot weather we add an additional quart. Dehydration is a common problem and can cause headaches, muscle aches, constipation, and weight gain. We take daily supplements of iodine, magnesium, and potassium. We season our food with sea salt which helps detox the body of bromine and fluorine.

If you decide to try a low carbohydrate diet we recommend reading Dr. Bruce Fife's book *The Coconut Ketogenic Diet* and Dr. Stephen Phinney's book *The Art and Science of Low Carbohydrate Performance*. Iodine supplements are also a key part of our improved metabolism, weight loss, and ability to stay off caffeine. If you are considering iodine supplements, we recommend reading Dr David Brownstein's book *Iodine: Why you need it; Why you can't live without it.*

The Institute of Medicine recommends an hour of moderately intense physical activity.[1] But we have found that 30 to 45 minutes of moderate physical activity keeps us in better shape. Our experience with intense workouts was that they make us overly tired, hungry, and sore. We have found that consistency and enjoyment of exercise is far more important than intensity for long term results.

During our long journey to health and weight loss in Hawaii, we tried many different approaches. Ultimately the diet and activities that allowed us to achieve our weight and health goals have become our overall approach to life.

References

1. Institute of Medicine of the National Academies, "Dietary Reference Intakes for Energy Carbohydrate, Fiber, Fat, Fatty Acids, Cholesterol, Protein, and Amino Acids," Released September 5, 2002, report available online: http://www.iom.edu/Reports/2002/Dietary-Reference-Intakes-for-Energy-Carbohydrate-Fiber-Fat-Fatty-Acids-Cholesterol-Protein-and-Amino-Acids.aspx last accessed 12/1/2014.
2. Jeff Volek and Stephen Phinney, *The Art and Science of Low Carbohydrate Performance* (Beyond Obesity LLC 2011)
3. Stephen Phinney, "Ketogenic diets and physical performance," *Nutrition & Metabolism* 1, no 1 (2004): 1-2.
4. David Brownstein, *Iodine: Why you need it; Why you can't live without it,* 5th Edition (Michigan: Medical Alternatives Press 2014)
5. Fife, Bruce, *The Coconut Ketogenic Diet* (Colorado Springs: Piccadilly Books 2014)

<u>OUTLINE OF OUR HAWAII DIET</u>

- **<u>Light</u>** - We get daily exposure to sunlight of at least 500 Lux for 15 to 30 minutes, preferably early in the day.

- **<u>Iodine</u>** –We get daily exposure to the ocean mist and eat fish. We avoid bromine, fluorine, and other iodine inhibitors when possible. After reading Dr. David Brownstein's book, *Iodine: Why you need it; Why you can't live without it* we started taking iodine supplements as well.

- **<u>Water</u>**: - We drink filtered, alkaline water and try to keep our body in an alkaline state to lower the chances of cancer or other chronic diseases in our bodies.

- **<u>Saturated Fat</u>** –We eat at least 60% fat from coconut oil and animals fats. We avoid all vegetable and seed oils.

- **<u>Protein</u>** –We limit our protein consumption in meat, fish, and eggs to 25% of our daily calories.

- **Carbohydrates** –We eat 50 grams or less of carbohydrates daily (200 calories) to keep in nutritional ketosis. We eat no grains, no sugar, and limit our fructose.

- **Physical Activity** –We exercise 30 to 45 minutes a day with moderate walking, swimming, water aerobics, or other physical activity. We are outside in nature every day.

- **Fun** – We make time to have fun, learn new things, and appreciate our life every day.

WHAT WE EAT AND DRINK

- Water: We drink at least one quart of water for every 60 pounds of bodyweight each day.
- Saturated Fat: We cook with coconut oil and animal fats and we avoid vegetable and seed oils.
- Meat: We eat beef, pork, chicken, and turkey. We are lucky to have nearby ranches that raise grass-fed cattle. We count the grams of protein.
- Fish: We eat local, canned, and frozen ocean fish. We avoid farm-

raised fish. We count the grams of protein.

- <u>Dairy</u>: We eat eggs, cheese, cottage cheese, and plain yoghurt. We count the grams of protein and carbohydrates.
- <u>Nuts</u>: We eat macadamia nuts, almonds, pecans and other tree nuts in moderation. We avoid peanuts and cashews which are not nuts. We count the grams of protein and carbohydrates.
- <u>Low-carbohydrate vegetables</u>: We eat low carbohydrate vegetables such as celery, cucumbers, lettuce, mushrooms, parsley, peppers, radishes, artichokes, asparagus, avocados, bamboo shoots, broccoli, brussels sprouts, cabbage, cauliflower, swiss chard, collard greens, eggplant, green string beans, hearts of palm, kale, leeks, okra, olives, onions, pumpkin, sauerkraut, snow peas, spinach, tomatoes, turnips, and water chestnuts. We buy organic when possible. We count the carbohydrates in the vegetables.
- <u>Fruit</u>: We eat unsweetened blueberries, cherries, lemons, and limes. We only buy organic and we count the carbohydrates.

- <u>Alcohol:</u> We drink alcohol in moderation, 4 ounces a day or less
- <u>No caffeine:</u> We no longer drink coffee, energy drinks, tea, and try to avoid over-the-counter medicines with caffeine
- <u>Supplements</u>: We supplement our diet with Iodine (Lugols 2% solution – 12 to 25 mg a day), ATP Factors (B2 and B3), Magnesium, and Potassium.

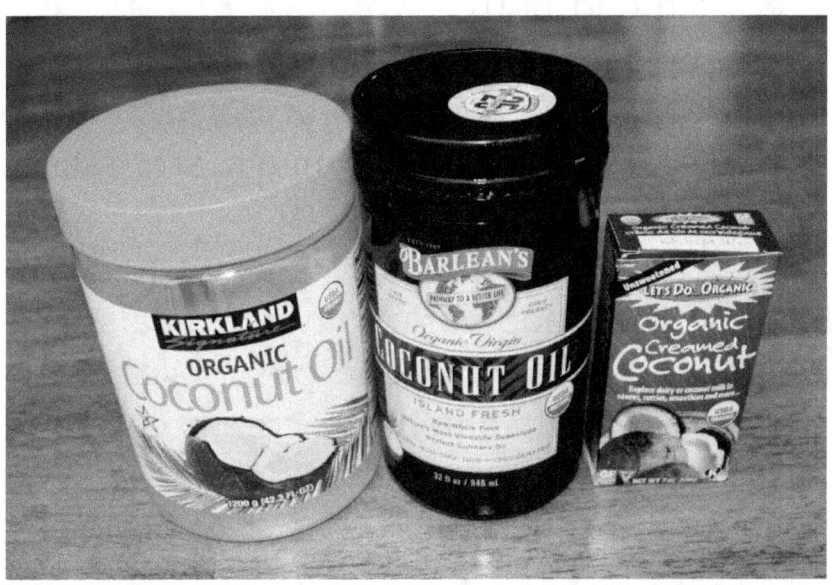

Coconut oil and creamed coconut products

Our diet is simple and repetitive. We have eggs and bacon for breakfast, meat for lunch, and a salad for dinner. We never tire of eggs and bacon for breakfast. Lunch is our major meal and we vary the seasonings and meat recipes including barbeques, stews, tuna melts, burgers (with no bun), and stir fry. Our salads consist of lettuce, tomatoes, coconut oil, topped with cheese, fish, or meat. We have a moderate amount of vegetables like broccoli, potatoes, V8 and others within the allotted daily carbohydrates.

We eat almond butter, yoghurt, or cottage cheese for a snack and often mix them with blueberries. A benefit of our coconut ketogenic diet is that our meals are easy to prepare.

We sometimes add variety in our meals by making a quiche or meat pie. We also make pumpkin or blueberry cream cheese pie for special occasions. Our pie crusts are made of ground nuts instead of grains.

We drink water throughout the day. We also enjoy herb tea, like peppermint tea, and wine in the evening.

By minimizing the carbohydrates we eat, we are able to remain in nutritional ketosis.

We are less hungry between meals and no longer have sudden weight gains if we eat or drink more than we planned. Best of all, we have greater stamina mentally and physically to accomplish the many goals we have set for ourselves.

INDEX

INDEX

Acknowledgements

We want to acknowledge our friends and family for their support and interest in our books. We thank everyone who bought our books and inspired us to continue to write about life in Hawaii. We thank Bob Dempsey for insisting our next book answer the mystery of why people in Hawaii are so healthy. Studying this question turned out to be a blessing to our health and we hope others find our research helpful in improving their health.

We thank Bill Hodges for listening to Tyler try and explain what he was learning in the health studies and Lois Hodges for all her support and invaluable help proofreading this book. We thank Bob and Marilyn Puschinsky for patiently listening to our diet insights. Paul Carr endured content testing and we thank him for his time and interest. We also thank Kim Dempsey and Bill and Shirley Fritz for their support. Every conversation we had with our friends helped us write the book.

We thank our son Daniel for his enthusiastic support of this research project and for our countless evenings of lively discussion with him about our research. His support extended to being willing to change his diet to try out our health discoveries and help verify they really do work.

We thank Joy and Brenda at Kona Stories for providing an amazing bookstore in Kona. We thank our parents David, Tish, and Jackie for their constant support.

About the Authors

Tyler and Chris Mercier moved to Hawaii Island to slow down from their fast-paced life in Silicon Valley. Since 2007, they have lived in Hilo, Kailua-Kona, and Kamuela where they experienced living in different homes, communities, and climate zones on the island. Tyler and Chris write books, blogs, and websites about homes, health, local foods, and the tropical lifestyle on Hawaii Island.

The Mercier's blog at hiloliving.blogspot.com
Their websites are:
hiloliving.com
hawaiihealthy.com
youridealhawaii.com

Other books by Tyler and Chris Mercier:
Your Ideal Hawaii Island Vacation: A Guide for Visiting the Big Island of Hawaii
Your Ideal Hawaii Day Planner
Your Ideal Hawaii Island Move: A Guide for Moving to Hawaii Island
Your Ideal Hawaii Home: Avoid Disaster when Buying or Building in Hawaii

The authors can be contacted at
youridealhawaii@gmail.com